Occupational Therapy and Physical Therapy: A Resource and Planning Guide
Second Edition

Developed by
Patricia Bober, MS, OT
Occupational Therapy Consultant
Wisconsin Department of Public Instruction

Sandra Corbett, PT
Physical Therapy Consultant
Wisconsin Department of Public Instruction

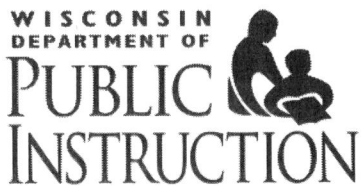

Wisconsin Department of Public Instruction
Tony Evers, PhD, State Superintendent
Madison, Wisconsin

This publication is available from:

Wisconsin Department of Public Instruction
125 South Webster Street
Madison, WI 53703
608/266-2188
http://dpi.wi.gov/sped/tm-specedtopics.html

Bulletin No. 1106

ISBN 978-1-57337-148-3

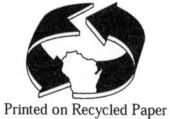

Printed on Recycled Paper

Foreword

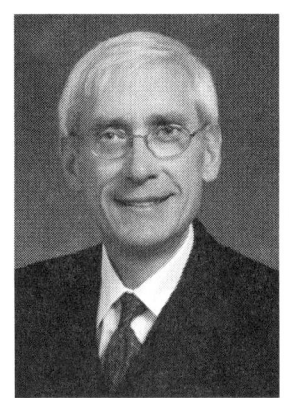

Occupational therapists and physical therapists have provided services to children in Wisconsin's schools for almost 40 years. Their role is to help children develop skills and perform tasks that most people take for granted in their own lives.

The Department of Public Instruction created this book to explain how occupational therapists (OTs) and physical therapists (PTs) collaborate with educators, administrators, and parents to support the mission of education in the environment of the schools. This book answers questions about who OTs and PTs are, what their purpose is in schools, and how, working with educators and parents, they help Wisconsin's children acquire the skills and knowledge they need to participate alongside other children in school and, eventually, assume positive adult roles in the community.

This publication will help school staff and parents better understand the key roles OTs and PTs play in the lives of children who need their services to benefit from their education. Their work supports our shared goal that every child will graduate with the knowledge and skills needed to be successful in the workforce and/or higher education. I believe this publication will support the work of all of us who believe education is the most important element to ensure a successful future for our children and our nation.

Tony Evers
State Superintendent

Acknowledgments

The authors wish to thank all the occupational therapists, physical therapists, occupational therapy assistants, physical therapist assistants, and special educators in Wisconsin who asked the questions that led to the development of this resource and planning guide. The following people provided help and support in many ways: by writing and reviewing drafts; by sharing materials; and by providing feedback and encouragement.

Kris Barnekow, Ph.D., OTR
University of Illinois
Chicago, Illinois

Valerie D. Clevenger, PT, MS, PCS
Waunakee School District
Waunakee, Wisconsin

Judy Dewane, PT, MHS, NCS
University of Wisconsin
Madison, Wisconsin

Lori Dominiczak, PT, MS
Dominiczak Therapy Associates, LLC
Brown Deer, Wisconsin

Marie Dorie
Director of Special Ed/Pupil Services
CESA 2
Milton, Wisconsin

Mardi Freeman
Director of Special Education and Pupil Services
Hamilton School District
Sussex, Wisconsin

Kerry Gloss, OTR
Green Bay Public Schools
Green Bay, Wisconsin

Gerry Heuer, BS, COTA
DeForest School District
DeForest, Wisconsin

Dan Kutschera, PT
Neenah School District
Neenah, Wisconsin

Marcia Obukowicz, OT
CESA 9
Tomahawk, Wisconsin

Tracy Prill, OTA
Edgerton School District
Edgerton, Wisconsin

Lisa Pugh
Parent
Madison, Wisconsin

Judy Schabert, OTR
Salucare Rehabilitation Service
LaCrosse, Wisconsin

Kathy Tomczyk, PTA, MS
Milwaukee Area Technical College
Milwaukee, Wisconsin

Patty Weynand, PT
Madison Metropolitan School District
Madison, Wisconsin

Janesville School District
Janesville, Wisconsin

Waukesha School District
Waukesha, Wisconsin

Special thanks to:

Division for Learning Support: Equity and Advocacy

Carolyn Stanford Taylor, Assistant State Superintendent
Stephanie Petska, Director, Special Education Team

State Superintendent's Office

Meri Annin, Education Information Services
Kari Gensler Santistevan, Education Information Services

Margaret T. Dwyer, Editor

Copyrighted Materials

Every effort has been made to ascertain proper ownership on copyrighted materials and to obtain permission for this use. Any omission is unintentional.

Table of Contents

Introduction

Occupational Therapy and Physical Therapy: A Resource and Planning Guide, Second Edition

This book, *Occupational Therapy and Physical Therapy: A Resource and Planning Guide, Second Edition*, defines and explains the meaning and purpose of these interrelated, but distinct, types of therapy and offers readers the opportunity to understand the roles of therapists as part of the school environment. Readers may wish to read the entire book as a whole, or may choose to focus on those chapters or sections most related to their work. Every chapter is understandable on its own, but a complete reading will result in more comprehensive and effective understanding for the reader. A revision of the first edition published in 1996, the book is thoroughly updated to reflect the changing practice of school-based therapies.

This book explains the work and roles of occupational therapists and physical therapists in Wisconsin's schools.

Chapter 1 provides basic historical information to readers about occupational therapy and physical therapy with children in schools. The chapter introduces a collaborative model of service that subsequent chapters describe in greater depth.

Chapter 2 offers succinct descriptions and interpretations of the state and federal laws that apply to occupational therapy and physical therapy in the schools. As part of this, the chapter covers recent changes in licensure and certification issues that all occupational therapists (OTs) and physical therapists (PTs) should know.

In chapter 3, readers gain access to the two initial steps of therapy: eligibility and process. Process involves recognizing the need to evaluate a child for occupational therapy or physical therapy, planning a program that includes either therapy, and delivering services that maximize outcomes most useful to the child in school. The third chapter also features many tools to help educators and therapists understand their roles in the process. Sample checklists will assist teachers in describing the performance of a child who needs strategies or accommodations. In addition, these tools allow teachers to record previous efforts made in response to the child's needs. A sample Individualized Education Program resulting from a team evaluation contains a variety of helpful, detailed examples of goals and objectives that occupational therapy or physical therapy supports.

Chapter 4 focuses specifically on occupational therapy and the role of the OTs in schools. Both the text and figures of this chapter clarify the purpose of occupational therapy: the support of health and participation in life through engagement in occupation. The authors present and use conceptual frameworks to discuss the critical elements of occupational therapy practice. The chapter ends with a brief discussion of the ethics of the profession.

In chapter 5, the focus shifts to physical therapy and the particular role of the PT in the schools. The chapter's graphics and narrative explain physical therapy's concentration on motor function, paying special attention to the impact of mobility and functional movement on the child's participation in classroom and school activities. As in the chapter before it, chapter 5 includes an overview of the profession's ethics.

Chapter 6 describes service provision when a supervisory relationship exists among therapy personnel. The chapter addresses supervision requirements in state law. Such personnel include licensed therapists, licensed assistants, student therapists, and school staff who are not licensed in the fields of occupational therapy or physical therapy.

Collaboration is the central idea of chapter 7, which stresses communication and ongoing understanding among professionals and with parents. In comparison to various models of service delivery, the collaborative model remains the most effective within school systems. Chapter 7 delves into the need to recognize the ongoing changes that children, educators, therapists, and parents all undergo, and the need for strong communication so that services are neither overlooked nor needlessly repeated. Directors of special education are the individuals responsible for overseeing the delivery of these services, and chapter 8 presents issues and information relevant to them. This chapter is filled with helpful sample forms, including staff performance appraisals, workload estimations, and those that will help administrators better understand and supervise related service providers. This eighth chapter also will help administrators support the collaboration and communication presented in chapter 7.

The book concludes with the question and answer format of Chapter 9. This chapter helps the reader revisit the most frequent issues that involve occupational therapy or physical therapy. Whether readers begin or end their reading of this guide with chapter 9, they will find succinct answers to the tougher questions that parents, teachers, school therapists, and administrators ask the authors about occupational therapy or physical therapy every day.

Finally, the book's appendices support and supplement the nine text chapters that precede them. Contact information for agencies and other organizations, sample treatment plans, codes of ethics for both occupational therapy and physical therapy, resources that describe roles and activities of school-based therapists, and forms for safe use of equipment all appear in this last section to explain and enhance the work of OTs and PTs in Wisconsin's schools.

Readers will find succinct answers to the tougher questions that parents, teachers, school therapists, and administrators ask every day.

Occupational Therapy and Physical Therapy in Wisconsin Schools

1

Prior to 1973, occupational therapists (OTs) and physicals therapists (PTs) treated children primarily in medical facilities; medically oriented residential facilities; and separate educational facilities for children with disabilities, commonly known as orthopedic schools. These facilities, while representing advancement in the provision of services to children, were separate from the educational and community environments that most children without disabilities experienced. Through the early 1970s, occupational therapy and physical therapy were deeply rooted in a medical orientation where both professionals and laypeople perceived individuals with disabilities as either continually sick or able to be *fixed.* (Rainforth and York-Barr, 1997) The training and preparation of OTs and PTs, in association with medical education overall, sustained the practice of focusing on factors within the patient or client, and removing children from their routine environments for isolated treatment. These practices reflected the common assumption that treatment would result in improved skills that would generalize to everyday life.

In 1973, Wisconsin law established OTs and PTs as members of the multidisciplinary teams who served children with exceptional educational needs in public schools. Many OTs and PTs needed to shift their emphasis from success within the special education environment to a different model. The traditional approach of minimizing the effect of a physical disability or handicapping condition and measuring performance only by testing needed to be replaced. The medical model of isolated treatment sessions, most of which took place away from children's classrooms, no longer met the needs of school systems focused on involvement and participation.

The Changing Practice of School Therapy

As best educational practices evolved to support the integration of children with disabilities in all aspects of school and community life, the practices of occupational therapy and physical therapy in school changed. Schools today continue to emphasize providing services and supports in general education environments and increasing collaboration among educational team members. In addition, the active involvement of parents and individuals with disabilities in decision making, in combination with many years of literature in special education and related services supports this emphasis.

A collaborative model that includes OTs, PTs, general educators, special educators, and parents looks very different than an expert model rooted in a traditional medical orientation. An expert consultant expects to have answers to people's questions, and protects his or her domain of knowledge and strategies. In collaborative consultation, team members work together to solve problems by sharing information, coordinating activities, and teaching strategies to other team members. Appropriateness and usefulness of joint action drives the joint decision making. Researchers have found that because educators prefer the collaborative consultation model, they implement more of the consultant's recommendations than when consultants use other models. (Babcock and Pryzwanski, 1983)

A collaborative model does not exclude the provision of direct service by OTs and PTs. It simply places their specific techniques into a larger framework of functional outcomes in real environments, determined by team decision-making and evidence. When the first edition of this guide was published in 1996, evidence-based practice was just emerging in the professions of occupational therapy and physical therapy. It resembles both its predecessor, evidence-based medicine, and the research-based educational practices defined in the 2004 Individuals with Disabilities Education Act. In evidence-based practice, professionals review published research to gather the most reliable evidence about the effectiveness of selected interventions or practice patterns, and apply that evidence along with their own experience and reasoning to identify effective interventions for a specific client. (Law & Baum, 1998) Combined with the early and frequent measurement of an individual child's response to interventions, evidence-based practice is changing the way that school therapy is provided.

The authors of this guide apply the collaborative model of providing evidence-based related services in the least restrictive environment to the information here, focusing on the needs of therapists and administrators, while making the language and structure accessible to parents and educators as well. The success of this guide rests not only in its ability to serve as a resource, but also as a tool to generate discussion and improved communication among those who serve children with disabilities.

Schools today continue to emphasize providing services and supports in general education environments and increasing collaboration among educational team members.

References

Babcock, N.L. and W.B. Pryzwanski. 1983. "Models of Consultation: Preferences of Educational Professionals at Five Stages of Service." *School Psychology* 21: 359-366.

Law, M. and C. Baum. 1998. "Evidence-based Occupational Therapy." *Canadian Journal of Occupational Therapy* 65: 131-135.

Rainforth, B., and J. York-Barr. 1997. *Collaborative Teams for Students with Severe Disabilities 2nd edition.* Baltimore: Paul H. Brookes.

Federal Regulations and State Rules

2

Federal statutes and regulations, as well as state statutes and administrative rules, regulate school-based occupational therapy and school-based physical therapy. Federal special education law is found in the Individuals with Disabilities Education Act (IDEA) and in Federal Regulations 34 CFR Part 300. State special education law in Wisconsin is found in Subchapter V, Chapter 115 of the Wisconsin Statutes (Wis. Stats.), and in Chapter PI 11 of the Wisconsin Administrative Code (Wis. Admin Code). These laws address occupational therapy and physical therapy as part of special education and related services in schools. Other state statute and administrative rules further regulate the practice of occupational therapy and physical therapy, regardless of where in Wisconsin a therapist practices. Chapter 448, Wis. Stats., subchapter VII regulates occupational therapy licensure and practice and subchapter III regulates physical therapy licensure and practice. Wis. Admin Code, Chapters OT 1 through 5 regulate occupational therapy and Chapters PT 1 through 9 regulate physical therapy. Internet links to specific legislation appear at the end of this chapter.

Federal special education law is found in the Individuals with Disabilities Education Act and in Federal Regulations.

Individuals with Disabilities Education Act (IDEA)

IDEA is the federal law that governs the education of children with disabilities. One of the purposes of IDEA is to ensure all children with disabilities have available a free, appropriate public education that emphasizes special education and related services designed to meet their unique needs and prepare them for further education, employment, and independent living. Another purpose is to ensure that the rights of children with disabilities and their families are protected. Six key principles of IDEA are free, appropriate public education, appropriate evaluation, an individualized education program, a least restrictive environment, parent and student participation in decision making, and procedural safeguards.

1. Free appropriate public education (FAPE) means that special education and related services are

   - free and at no cost to parents.

   - appropriate to the individual needs of the child.

   - publicly provided and funded.

   - educational, including academic, nonacademic and extra-curricular activities.

2. Appropriate evaluation means gathering information related to enabling the child to both be involved and progress in the general education

curriculum. For preschool children, an appropriate evaluation means gathering information related to allowing the child to participate in appropriate activities. An appropriate evaluation ensures a student is not subjected to unnecessary tests and assessments.

3. Individualized education program (IEP) development is a collaborative process that occurs in a meeting and results in a document. The IEP document states the special education and related services the district will provide for the student.

4. Least restrictive environment (LRE) means that to the maximum extent appropriate, children with disabilities and children without disabilities are educated together. Special classes, separate schooling, or other removal of children with disabilities from the regular educational environment occurs only if the nature or severity of the disability is such that, even with the use of supplementary aids and services, education in regular classes cannot be achieved satisfactorily. IEP teams start with considering placement in regular classes in the neighborhood school. School districts must offer a continuum of alternative placements to meet the special education and related service needs of children with disabilities. IEP teams must explain in the IEP the extent to which the child will not participate with nondisabled children in academic, nonacademic and extracurricular activities.

5. Parent and student participation in decision making means parents participate equally on the IEP team in all phases and, in Wisconsin, students 14 years or older must be invited to IEP team meetings. A district must tell parents what it is going to do, or refuse to do, before it does so, and why.

6. Procedural safeguards ensure that the rights of children with disabilities and the rights of their parents are protected, that children with disabilities and their parents are provided with the information they need to make decisions about FAPE, and that procedures and mechanisms are in place to resolve disagreements between parties. An IEP team works toward reaching consensus about the education program for the child. When parents and the school disagree, there are formal ways to solve problems which include

   - independent educational evaluation (IEE).
   - facilitated IEP.
   - mediation.
   - IDEA complaint.
   - due process hearing.

Procedural safeguards ensure that the rights of children with disabilities and the rights of their parents are protected.

IDEA contains requirements for the evaluation of a child suspected of having a disability and for the development of an IEP. These requirements, as they relate to school occupational therapists (OTs) and school physical therapists (PTs), receive more attention in subsequent chapters of this guide. This chapter and the brief definitions that follow allow readers to confirm their understanding of the fundamental terms of special education used in the context of this book.

Special education refers to the instruction that a team of school staff and parents specially design to meet the unique needs of a child with a disability, and which the school provides at no cost to parents. It may include instruction in the classroom, in physical education, at home, in hospitals, in institutions, and in other settings. A child's special education program incorporates the services of a licensed special education teacher, or a physical education teacher in the case of specially designed physical education, to implement the IEP. More information about specially designed physical education is in *DPI Information Update Bulletin 10.04 Physical Education for Children with Disabilities.* (2010) In Wisconsin, speech and language services are regarded as special education or as related services as determined appropriate by the IEP team.

Related services are those required to assist a child with a disability to benefit from special education. IDEA specifically includes occupational therapy and physical therapy as related services.

Section 504 of the Rehabilitation Act

IDEA is not the only federal law that addresses the education of children with disabilities. Section 504 of the Rehabilitation Act of 1973, a civil rights law, protects the rights of individuals with disabilities and prohibits discrimination on the basis of disability in any program or activity receiving federal financial assistance. (34 CFR sec.104.1) State education agencies (SEAs) and local educational agencies (LEAs) such as school districts, Cooperative Educational Service Agencies (CESAs) and County Children with Disabilities Education Boards (CCDEBs) receive federal funding and must meet the requirements of the act. Section 504 covers a qualified student with a disability when the student has a physical or mental impairment which substantially limits one or more of the major life activities, has a record of such an impairment, or is regarded as having such an impairment. (34 CFR sec. 104.3 (j) (1))

The regulation defines physical or mental impairment as "(a) any physiological disorder or condition, cosmetic disfigurement, or anatomical loss affecting one or more of the following body systems: neurological; musculoskeletal; special sense organs; respiratory, including speech organs; cardiovascular; reproductive, digestive, genitourinary; hemic and lymphatic; skin; and endocrine; or (b) any mental or psychological disorder, such as mental retardation, organic brain syndrome, emotional or mental illness, and specific learning disabilities." (34 CFR s. 104.3 (j) (2) (i))

Congress expanded the definition of major life activities with amendments effective January 1, 2009. Major life activities include but are not limited to

Section 504 protects the rights of individuals with disabilities and prohibits discrimination on the basis of disability in any program or activity receiving federal financial assistance.

caring for oneself, performing manual tasks, seeing, hearing, eating, sleeping, walking, standing, lifting, bending, speaking, breathing, learning, reading, concentrating, thinking, communicating, and working. A major life activity also includes the operation of a major bodily function, including but not limited to functions of the immune system, normal cell growth, digestive, bowel, bladder, neurological, brain, respiratory, circulatory, endocrine and reproductive functions. An impairment that substantially limits one major life activity need not limit other major life activities in order to be considered a disability. An impairment that is episodic or in remission is a disability if it would substantially limit a major life activity when active. For example, a student with a seizure disorder that is in remission would meet this requirement.

An LEA may not factor into the decision making the impact of mitigating measures when determining the existence of a disability. Mitigating measures include medication, medical supplies, equipment, appliances, low-vision devices, prosthetics including limbs and devices, hearing aids and cochlear implants or implantable hearing devices, mobility devices, or oxygen therapy equipment and supplies; use of assistive technology; reasonable accommodations or auxiliary aids or services; or learned behavioral or adaptive neurological modifications. (34 CFR s.104.3(j) (2) (ii)) Although the ameliorating affects of these measures, with the exception of eyeglasses and contact lenses, may have a positive impact, they do not remove or cancel out the existence of the disability. For example, school districts cannot consider the effect of medication on a student with asthma, and rule out the disability that asthma produces.

In public schools a qualified student with a disability under Section 504 must have access to public school programs and activities, and no one has the right to subject the student to discrimination. In addition, Section 504 requires public schools to provide FAPE to each qualified student with a disability. Section 504 requires recipients of federal funding to provide students with disabilities appropriate educational services designed to meet the individual needs of such students. Their needs should be met to the same extent as the needs of students without disabilities are met. Under Section 504 regulations, an appropriate education for a student with a disability could include education in regular classrooms, education in regular classes with supplementary services, and special education and related services. Section 504 also compels schools to conduct an appropriate evaluation; determine eligibility through a group of persons, including persons knowledgeable about the meaning of the evaluation data and knowledgeable about placement options; conduct periodic reevaluations; and establish and implement procedural safeguards. Compliance with the procedures and requirements described in IDEA is one way of meeting the requirements of Section 504.

A student who does not qualify for services under IDEA may qualify for services under Section 504. A qualified student will have what is commonly called a *504 plan* or an *accommodation plan*. The plan states the accommodations, aids, or services the student will receive. Occupational therapy or physical therapy may be in a student's accommodation plan. The individual student's

A student who does not qualify for services under IDEA may qualify for services under Section 504.

needs determine the amount of therapy, and it is not limited to indirect service or consultation. School districts identify a Section 504 coordinator to respond to referrals. If additional information is necessary, the Department of Education, Office for Civil Rights, and not the Wisconsin Department of Public Instruction (DPI), is the next point of reference. Appendix A, *Organizations*, under *Federal Agencies* lists contact information for the Office for Civil Rights. A list of frequently asked questions about Section 504 may be found at http://www.ed.gov/about/offices/list/ocr/504faq.html.

Subchapter V, Chapter 115, Wisconsin Statutes

In Wisconsin, Subchapter V, Chapter 115 of the Wisconsin statutes and the administrative code that implements it, Chapter PI 11, guarantee that children with disabilities receive appropriate services. As in the federal law, Wisconsin law requires school districts to provide children with disabilities with FAPE, which includes special education and related services. These services must be provided under public supervision and direction and without charge to parents. The services must conform to statutes and rules enforced by DPI and must be provided in conformity with a child's IEP.

IEP Team

Under Wisconsin law, public schools and other agencies have specific responsibilities to identify children and youth who may have disabilities. The school district appoints an IEP team of individuals to conduct an evaluation of the child. Except for the child's parent, these individuals must be employed by or under contract with the district. IEP team members must include

The school district appoints an IEP team of individuals to conduct an evaluation of the child.

- the parents of the child.

- at least one regular education teacher if the child is or may be participating in a regular educational environment.

- at least one special education teacher who has recent training or experience related to the child's known or suspected area of special education needs or, where appropriate, at least one special education provider of the child.

- an LEA representative who is qualified to provide or supervise the provision of special education, is knowledgeable about the general education curriculum, and is knowledgeable about and authorized to commit the available resources of the LEA.

- an individual who can interpret the instructional implications of evaluation results.

- other participants who have knowledge or special expertise regarding the child at the discretion of the parent or the LEA.

- the child whenever appropriate.

- a representative of the child's district of residence when the child is attending school in a nonresident school district.

An IEP team must include an OT if the child is suspected of needing occupational therapy and a PT if the child is suspected of needing physical therapy. (Ch. P1 11.24(2), Wis. Admin Code) The district must obtain written consent from the child's parent before it can conduct an initial IEP team evaluation that includes occupational therapy or physical therapy.

Members of the IEP team assess specific areas of educational need using valid, appropriate, and non-discriminatory evaluation procedures. The special education director or case manager schedules an IEP team meeting to discuss the members' evaluations, findings, and other relevant data. Using the criteria in the state rule, the IEP team must determine if the child has an impairment as listed in Figure 1 and whether the child needs special education. Criteria for each of the impairment areas are specified in Chapter PI 11.36, Wis. Admin Code. When determining the child's need for special education, the team may consider these questions:

- Does the student have needs that cannot be met in the regular education program as it is currently structured?

- Are there modifications such as adaptation of content, methodology, or delivery of instruction that can be made in the regular education program to allow the student access to the general education curriculum?

- Could these modifications allow the student to meet the educational standards of instruction?

- What modifications do not require special education?

- What modifications do require special education?

- Are there additions or modifications such as replacement content, expanded core curriculum, or other supports the child needs that are not provided through the general education curriculum?

If the child has an impairment and needs special education, the child is a child with a disability. Figure 2 represents an overall perspective and basic chronology of the IEP team process.

The IEP team must determine if the child has an impairment and whether the child needs special education.

Figure 1 Impairment Areas

Autism

Cognitive Disability

Emotional Behavioral Disability

Hearing Impairment

Orthopedic Impairment

Other Health Impairment

Significant Developmental Delay

Specific Learning Disability

Speech or Language Impairment

Traumatic Brain Injury

Visual Impairment

Figure 2 IEP Team Process

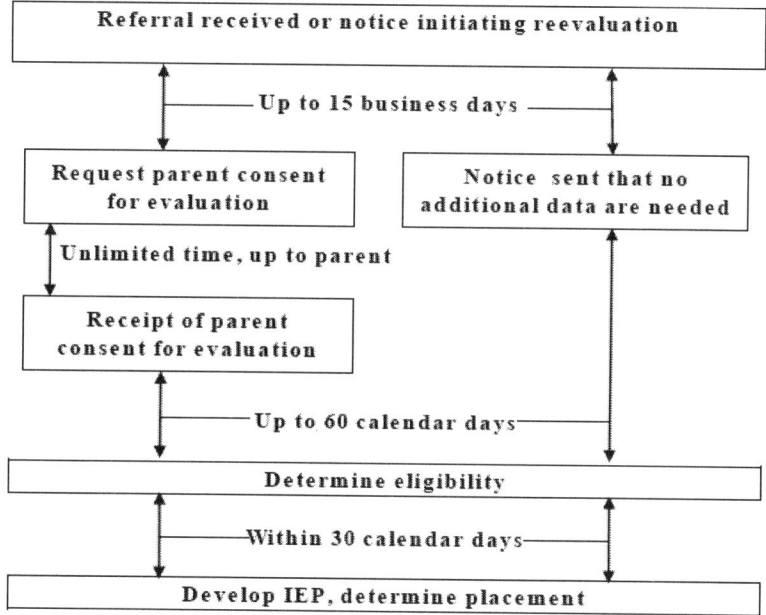

Individualized Education Program

Each child receiving special education services under IDEA or Wisconsin law must have an IEP. The IEP team develops the IEP and determines placement. The IEP reflects the written commitment of the district to the resources necessary to enable a child with a disability to receive needed special education and related services. It specifies or provides

The IEP reflects the written commitment of the district to the resources necessary to enable a child with a disability to receive needed special education and related services.

- information about the child's present level of academic achievement and functional performance.

- measurable annual goals including short-term objectives or benchmarks for the student who takes alternate assessments.

- how the child's progress toward attaining annual goals will be measured and when periodic reports will be provided to the parents.

- the type of special education and related services to be provided, including assistive technology services or devices, if appropriate; supplementary aids and services; and program modifications and supports for school personnel.

- the amount, frequency, duration and location of services.

- the extent to which the child will not participate with nondisabled children in regular classes, curriculum, extracurricular and other nonacademic activities.

- a statement of measurable postsecondary goals and transition services if the child is fourteen years of age or older.

- a statement of any accommodations necessary on statewide or LEA-wide assessments, or a statement of why the child cannot participate in the regular assessment and why an alternate assessment is appropriate for the child.

Chapter PI 11.24, Wis. Admin Code addresses the provision of occupational therapy and physical therapy as related services. The components of this chapter are summarized in Figure 3.

Attending Meetings

The excusal provisions in IDEA permit any required member of the IEP team to be excused from attending the IEP team meeting, in whole or part, if the parent agrees in writing. As noted in Ch. PI 11.24(2), Wis. Admin Code, OTs and PTs are required members when the respective therapy is part of the child's current evaluation, reevaluation or IEP. If therapists cannot attend an IEP team meeting

Figure 3 Occupational Therapy and Physical Therapy Rules Summary

IEP Team. If a child is suspected of needing occupational therapy or physical therapy or both, the IEP team includes the appropriate therapist.

Responsibilities of the Therapist. The therapist conducts all therapy evaluations and reevaluations for the child, participates in the development of the child's IEP, and develops the treatment plan for the child. An assistant cannot represent a therapist on an IEP team.

Licensure. The occupational therapist, occupational therapy assistant, physical therapist, and physical therapist assistant must hold licenses issued by the Department of Public Instruction. Qualifications are specified in PI 34.34 (14) (15) (16) (17).

Medical Information. A physician's referral is not required for occupational therapy or physical therapy. Medical information is required before a child receives occupational therapy. Medical information from a licensed physician is required before a child receives physical therapy.

Caseload. The minimum caseload for a 1.0 FTE occupational therapist or physical therapist is 15 children. The maximum caseload for a 1.0 FTE occupational therapist or physical therapist is 30 children. The maximum caseload for a 1.0 FTE occupational therapist or physical therapist with one or more assistants is 45 children. A caseload may vary due to

- frequency and duration of therapy specified in the child's IEP
- preparation time
- student related activities
- travel time
- number of evaluations

Delegation and Supervision. The physical therapist delegates and supervises the therapy provided by the physical therapist assistant. The occupational therapist delegates and supervises the therapy provided by the occupational therapy assistant.

- The therapist delegates only those portions of a child's therapy which are consistent with the assistant's education, training, and experience.
- The therapist develops a written policy and procedure for written and oral communication to the assistant which includes a specific description of the supervisory activities undertaken for the assistant at either of these levels:

  Close Supervision. The therapist has daily, direct contact on the premises with the assistant.

  General Supervision. The therapist has direct face-to-face contact with the assistant at least once every 14 calendar days. The therapist provides on-site re-evaluation of each child's therapy a minimum of one time per calendar month or every tenth day of therapy, whichever is sooner, and adjusts the therapy plan as appropriate.

- In between direct contacts, the therapist is available by telecommunication.
- The therapist supervises no more than three assistants. A 1.0 FTE therapist may supervise no more than 2.0 FTE assistants. Ratios are prorated according to the FTE of the therapist.

Source: Chapter PI 11.24, Wisconsin Administrative Code

they must follow the excusal provisions to be absent. One provision allows a therapist to be absent when occupational therapy or physical therapy will not be discussed or changed. If the meeting does involve modification to or discussion of occupational therapy or physical therapy, another provision allows the respective therapist to submit written input into the development of the IEP before the meeting. OTs and PTs who participate in the development of an IEP may not cancel therapy for other children in order to attend an IEP Team meeting. A scheduling system that allows another therapist or assistant of the same discipline to provide therapy to the children while the therapist attends a meeting offers a solution.

OTs and PTs who participate in the development of an IEP may not cancel therapy for other children in order to attend an IEP Team meeting.

An occupational therapy assistant (OTA) or a physical therapist assistant (PTA) cannot represent a therapist at the IEP team meeting, because the scope of an assistant's training does not cover the interpretation of evaluation results for the purpose of determining the existence of a disability, the need for special education and related services, and programming. The assistant may contribute to program planning by communicating information about the child to the therapist. Because the therapist and assistant communicate at regular intervals, seldom would it be necessary for both the therapist and the assistant to attend the meeting. After the annual IEP review and revision, changes in the IEP can be made by either the whole IEP team through an IEP team meeting or by agreement between the parent and the school district. Parents receive a copy of the revised IEP and the school informs the IEP team and those responsible for implementation of the changes.

Chapter 3 describes the IEP in more detail. Chapter 4 elaborates on occupational therapy within the IEP team process, and chapter 5 describes the IEP team process specific to physical therapy.

Chapter 448, Wisconsin Statutes

Chapter 448, Wis. Stats., and the administrative code that implements it, OT 1 through 5, and PT 1 through 9, stipulate the licensure requirements and standards of practice for OTs, OTAs, PTs, and PTAs practicing in any setting in Wisconsin. These rules apply to school therapists except where PI 11.24, Wis. Admin Code, is more restrictive.

Occupational Therapy Practice Requirements

Chapters OT 1 through 5, Wis. Admin Code include standards of practice for occupational therapy. OTs and OTAs working in public schools must follow these standards, unless Chapter PI 11, Wis. Admin Code describes more restrictive standards. The following are key components of OT 4.

- If an OT or OTA provides evaluation or intervention in an educational environment, including the child's home, for children and youth with disabilities under IDEA or Section 504, the OT or OTA does not require a physician order or a referral from another health care provider.

- When conducting an evaluation, an OT considers the individual's medical, vocational, social, educational, family status, familial and personal goals, and includes an assessment of how occupational performance components and occupational performance contexts influence the individual's functional abilities and deficits in occupational performance areas.

- Evaluation methods may include observation, interviews, records review, and the use of structured or standardized evaluative tools or techniques.

- Evaluation results shall be documented in the individual's record and shall indicate the specific evaluation tools and methods used.

- The OT periodically evaluates the child's occupational performance areas and occupational performance components, documenting the results.

- The OT periodically and systematically reviews the effectiveness and efficacy of all aspects of the occupational therapy program.

- Upon discontinuation of occupational therapy, the OT compares the child's initial and current states of functional abilities and deficits in occupational performance areas and occupational performance components. The OT documents the results and prepares a discharge plan.

Evaluation methods may include observation, interviews, records review, and the use of structured or standardized evaluative tools or techniques.

Physical Therapy Practice Requirements

Chapter 448, Wis. Stats. and Chapters PT 1 through 9, Wis. Admin Code stipulate the requirements for PTs and PTAs practicing in any setting in Wisconsin. These rules apply to school therapists and assistants except where PI 11.24 rules are more restrictive, but Chapter PI 11, Wis. Admin Code *does not* address written referral and patient record, so it appears here in detail.

Written Referral

Under Chapter 448.56, Wis. Stats., a PT does not require a written referral from a physician to provide service in schools to children with disabilities. In addition, Chapter PT 6.01, Wis. Admin Code states "a written referral is not required to provide the following services, related to work, home, leisure, recreational and educational environments: conditioning, injury prevention and application of biomechanics, treatment of musculoskeletal injuries with the exception of acute fractures or soft tissue avulsions."

Patient Record

IDEA no longer requires that IEP team members submit an individual report for student evaluations. However, Chapter 448.56(5) Wis. Stats. requires that "a physical therapist shall create and maintain a patient record for every patient that physical therapist examines or treats." The statute is silent on what should be in the patient record. Professional documentation includes the following elements which would be part of the patient record:

- initial examination, including history, systems review, tests and measures, evaluation, diagnosis (impact of the condition on function), prognosis (predicted functional outcome), and plan of care

- re-examination to assess progress and modify interventions

- notes on interventions and response

- discharge summary (APTA 1999)

Licensure Requirements

A license from the Department of Regulation and Licensing (DRL) is required for all OTs, OTAs, PTs and PTAs who practice in Wisconsin including those who practice in Wisconsin schools. Individuals must renew the license every two years. DRL sends out notices for renewal when the license is about to expire. In addition, all occupational therapy and physical therapy staff must be licensed by the DPI to work in Wisconsin public schools.

Department of Regulation and Licensing

Wisconsin statutes require that a physical therapist shall create and maintain a patient record for every patient that physical therapist examines or treats.

The Occupational Therapists Affiliated Credentialing Board of Wisconsin (OTACB) licenses all OTs and OTAs practicing in Wisconsin. An individual who has graduated from an accredited occupational therapy program or an accredited occupational therapy assistant program and passed the examination administered by the National Board for Certification in Occupational Therapy (NBCOT) must complete an application from DRL and submit any required documentation in order to receive licensure from DRL as an OT or OTA. In some circumstances, DRL requires an oral examination. DRL may grant a temporary license to a new graduate waiting to take the NBCOT examination or waiting for the results, if that graduate practices under monthly consultation from a licensed OT until receiving the examination results. The DRL requires that license holders earn specific continuing education points during each two-year period. Occupational therapists may use the designation OT, and occupational therapy assistants may use the designation OTA if they hold DRL licenses. A person may not use the titles Occupational Therapist Registered (OTR) or Certified Occupational Therapy Assistant (COTA) unless they maintain current NBCOT certification; however, renewal of NBCOT certification is not required for continued licensure in Wisconsin.

The Physical Therapy Examining Board of Wisconsin (PTEB) licenses all PTs and PTAs practicing in Wisconsin. An individual who has graduated from a board-approved physical therapy or physical therapist assistant educational program must complete an application from DRL, submit the required documentation and pass a written examination, and in some circumstances, an oral examination, in order to receive a DRL license. DRL may grant a new graduate a temporary license if that graduate practices under the direct, immediate, and on premises supervision of a licensed PT until receiving the examination results. Figure 4 on page 18 covers the main points of DRL licensure requirements.

Department of Public Instruction

Chapter PI 34, Wis. Admin Code describes the requirements for licensure of school OTs, PTs, OTAs, and PTAs. These licenses are found in Subchapter XI – Additional Licenses. A DPI license lasts for five years. All licenses begin July 1 and end June 30 of the fifth year. DPI does not send out notices for renewal when the license is about to expire. An applicant for a DPI initial or renewal license must submit a photocopy of a current license from DRL. Figure 5 covers the main points of DPI licensure requirements. License applications and fees (currently $100) are found at http://dpi.wi.gov/tepdl/applications.html.

DPI is required by state law, s.118.19(10)(c), Wis. Stats. to conduct a criminal background check on every license applicant each time an application is submitted. Applicants who have lived, worked or physically attended college classes in a state other than Wisconsin after age 17 are required to submit fingerprints in order to conduct an FBI background check. Cards used for fingerprinting must be obtained directly from DPI unless the fingerprints will be prepared by the Central Milwaukee Police Department or Promissor (a private vendor). No other exceptions are made. After receiving the cards from DPI, the applicant must take them to a law enforcement agency to have prints taken. Options for fingerprinting are to

- phone DPI at 1-800-266-1027 and leave a fingerprint card request on the voice mail option, *request for application or fingerprint cards.*

- e-mail a request for cards to Educator Licensing by going to http://dpi.wi.gov/tepdl/licensing_mail.html. Requests must include the applicant's name and complete mailing address, as well as the six-digit DPI educator file number of applicants who previously held a Wisconsin educator license.

- obtain Inkless Fingerprinting by having prints prepared electronically by the private vendor, Promissor. Fingerprint cards are not required for this option. Services are offered at several sites in Wisconsin. An appointment can be made online on Promissor's website or by calling 1-888-204-6212. Detailed registration instructions and FAQs are at

  http://www.asisvcs.com/publications/pdf/fp5002.pdf.

Applicants who have lived, worked or physically attended college classes in a state other than Wisconsin after age 17 are required to submit fingerprints in order to conduct an FBI background check.

Figure 4 Department of Regulation and Licensing Requirements

	Written Exam	Oral Examination	Temporary License	License Renewal
Occupational Therapist	OTACB	In some circumstances	Granted to new graduates waiting to take NBCOT exam or learn results; requires monthly consultation under licensed OT.	Two-year license; 24 points of continuing education must be earned during each two-year period.
Occupational Therapy Assistant	OTACB	In some circumstances	Granted to new graduates waiting to take NBCOT exam or learn results; requires monthly consultation under licensed OT.	Two-year license; 24 points of continuing education must be earned during each two-year period.
Physical Therapist	PTEB	In some circumstances	Granted to new graduates waiting to take PTEB exam or learn results; requires direct, on-premise supervision by licensed PT.	Two-year license; 30 hours of continuing education must be earned during each two-year period.
Physical Therapist Assistant	PTEB	In some circumstances	Granted to new graduates waiting to take PTEB exam or learn results; requires direct, on-premise supervision by licensed PT.	Two-year license; 20 hours of continuing education must be earned during each two-year period.

Figure 5 DPI Licensure Requirements

DPI License Name and Number	Documentation Required	Application and Fee	Temporary License	Other
Occupational Therapist License 812 Occupational Therapy Assistant License 885 Physical Therapist License 817 Physical Therapist Assistant License 886	Photocopy of DRL license or submission of DRL license number from website	License application, form PI-1602-NP; fee as listed on form	One-year license if holding temporary DRL license	Five-year license; no additional continuing education required

Space and Facilities

OTs and PTs should discuss unique needs for space with the director of special education or pupil services or the district administrator. Although occupational therapy and physical therapy will frequently occur in the child's classroom, the therapy may require a separate space for evaluation, specialized treatment, and equipment storage. Access to a telephone, a computer, and hand washing facilities are also necessary.

The therapy may require a separate space for evaluation, specialized treatment, and equipment storage.

The Department of Commerce administers school building safety. The administrative rules for schools are found in Chapter Comm 78, Wis. Admin Code at http://www.legis.state.wi.us/rsb/code/comm/comm078.pdf. The Department of Health Services administers health codes which may be applicable to schools. These rules are found in Chapter DHS, Wis. Admin Code. Schools also follow applicable local safety and health codes and regulations. At the date of this book's publication, state codes and federal regulations that apply to health and safety in schools include

- Comm 78.01 regarding exits.

- Comm 78.02 regarding fire escapes.

- Comm 78.03 regarding stairways.

- Comm 78.04 regarding exit doors.

- Comm 78.05 regarding classrooms and floor space.

- Comm 78.06 regarding seats and desks.

- Comm 78.07 regarding fire extinguishers.

- Comm 78.08 regarding fire alarms.

- Comm 78.09 regarding heating plants.

- Comm 78.10 regarding sanitary equipment.

- 29 CFR s. 1910.1030 which implements the federal Occupational Safety and Health Administration standard to minimize employee exposure to blood-borne pathogens.

Questions about building regulations and codes may be directed to the Wisconsin Department of Commerce, 608-267-3606 or http://commerce.wi.gov/SB/SB-Div Contacts.html.

Laws Protecting Confidentiality

All records directly related to a student and maintained by the school district are pupil records. Federal and state laws provide specific protections to students and parents regarding pupil records. Federal definitions of pupil records are in the

Family Educational Rights and Privacy Act (FERPA). State statutes parallel federal definitions of pupil records and also specifically address patient health care records and pupil physical health records. Parents have the right to inspect and review the contents of their child's records; to request that the district amend the record's information if the parent believes the information is inaccurate, misleading, or violates the privacy or other rights of their child; and to know who besides themselves and authorized school personnel has access to this information. Disclosure of confidential information is limited to appropriate parties when necessary to implement educational laws or to protect the health or safety of the student or other individuals.

Chapter 146, Wis. Stats. includes OTs, PTs, OTAs, and PTAs under the definition of *health care provider*. Under this statute, all records a health care provider prepares or supervises related to the health of a patient, must remain confidential, released only with the informed consent of the parent or guardian. When a school district maintains patient health care records, it may release them to other school district employees without informed parental consent if access to those records is necessary to comply with a requirement in federal or state law, such as IDEA and Chapter 115, Wis. Stats., or if the employee is responsible for preparing or storing the records. But the parent maintains the right to know to whom information has been shared.

All records a health care provider prepares or supervises related to the health of a patient, must remain confidential, released only with the informed consent of the parent or guardian.

Health Information Privacy Accountability Act (HIPAA) provides protection for individually identifiable health information. Patient health care records maintained by schools are considered education records and are thus subject to FERPA rules and not the privacy portions of HIPAA. When school personnel want or need health information from outside health care providers, they must adhere to the disclosure requirements of the outside health care providers, which are HIPAA governed, in order to have access to the information. Schools that bill Wisconsin Medicaid electronically for school-based services should comply with transaction and code set standards of HIPAA for submission of electronic claims.

School districts develop their own local policies regarding student records and confidentiality based upon federal law and state statutes. DPI provides further guidance about student records and confidentiality in *Confidentiality of Records.* (2008) Chapter 8, Administration, provides more information about records.

References

34 CFR sec.104. http://www2.ed.gov/policy/rights/reg/ocr/edlite-34cfr104.html (accessed June 1, 2010).

American Physical Therapy Association. 1999. *Guide to Physical Therapist Practice.* Alexandria, VA: American Physical Therapy Association.

Wisconsin Department of Public Instruction. 2008. *Confidentiality of Records.* http://www.dpi.state.wi.us/sspw/pdf/srconfid.pdf (accessed June 1, 2010).

___. PI 11, Wis. Admin Code. http://www.dpi.state.wi.us/sped/pi11_0701.html (accessed June 1, 2010).

___. *Physical Education for Children with Disabilities*. 2010. http://dpi.wi.gov/sped/bul10-04.html (accessed September 10, 2010).

Other Resources

(accessed June 1, 2010).

Gamm, S. 2009. "Impact of the 2008 ADA Amendment on School Districts." Public Consulting Group. http://www.casecec.org/pdf/ADA%20Amendment%20Explanation%2012-14-08--Sue%20Gamm.pdf

U.S. Department of Education. IDEA 2004. http://idea.ed.gov/

Wisconsin Department of Commerce. http://www.legis.state.wi.us/rsb/code/comm/comm078.pdf

Wisconsin Department of Public Instruction. Home page. http://dpi.wi.gov/home.html

___. Eligibility Criteria. http://www.dpi.state.wi.us/sped/eligibility.html

___. *Least Restrictive Environment*. 2000. http://www.dpi.state.wi.us/sped/pdf/bul00-04.pdf

___. PI 34, Wis. Admin Code. http://dpi.wi.gov/tepdl/pi34.html#definitions3401

___. Section 504. http://www.dpi.state.wi.us/sped/sb504.html

___. Special Education Index. http://www.dpi.state.wi.us/sped/tm-specedtopics.html#e

___.Special Education Topics Reference. http://www.dpi.state.wi.us/sped/subjects.html#eval

Wisconsin Department of Regulation and Licensing. Home page. http://drl.wi.gov/index.asp?locid=0

___. Occupational Therapist and Occupational Therapy Assistant. http://drl.wi.gov/profession.asp?profid=28&locid=0

___. Physical Therapist and Physical Therapist Assistant.
http://drl.wi.gov/profession.asp?profid=37&locid=0

Wisconsin Legislature. Chapter 115, Wisconsin Statutes.
http://nxt.legis.state.wi.us/nxt/gateway.dll?f=templates&fn=default.htm&d=stats
&jd=ch.%20115

___. Chapter 448, Subchapter III, Wisconsin Statutes.
http://nxt.legis.state.wi.us/nxt/gateway.dll?f=templates&fn=default.htm&d=stats
&jd=448.50

The IEP Team Process in School

3

When a child has difficulty in school, teachers should identify the tasks and environments in which the child is not progressing or participating, try educational accommodations or interventions that they think will support the child, and monitor the child's response. This process is known as Response to Intervention (RtI) and is often part of a schoolwide system of coordinated early intervening services (CEIS) in general education. If a child is suspected of having a disability, teachers and parents may consider a special education evaluation and think about occupational therapy or physical therapy as related services to special education.

Referral

Teachers, parents, or any person who has reasonable cause to believe a child has a disability may refer the child for a special education evaluation. When parents or teachers suspect that a child may need occupational therapy or physical therapy, the IEP team for that child includes the appropriate therapist. The school district must initiate a special education initial evaluation or re-evaluation process if it is considering occupational therapy or physical therapy for a child. Occupational therapists (OTs) and physical therapists (PTs) should take an active role in helping teachers and special education directors determine when a child needs an occupational therapy or physical therapy evaluation. This may involve team discussions or staff in-services that focus on a better understanding of the roles of therapists in the educational setting. Therapists and teachers can work together to develop a checklist or reference sheet that traces the teacher's initial observations of a child's behavior, the interventions the teacher has attempted to meet the child's needs, the response to those interventions, and the reasons the teacher suspects a child needs an occupational therapy or physical therapy evaluation. Figures 6 and 7 on pages 26 and 27 are sample checklists that can serve as a guide for teachers when they are trying to determine whether or not to request an occupational therapy or physical therapy evaluation for a child.

The district must initiate a special education initial evaluation or re-evaluation process if it is considering occupational therapy or physical therapy for a child.

Initial Evaluation

The purpose of an initial evaluation is to determine a child's eligibility for special education and the educational needs of the child. The initial evaluation also gathers information related to

- enabling the child to be involved, as well as progress in the general education curriculum.

Figure 6 Sample Reference Guide for Teachers: Occupational Therapy

1. What are the environments in which I frequently observe the child? (Check ALL that apply.)
    - ❑ General classroom, large groups
    - ❑ Cafeteria or snack area
    - ❑ Recess or playground
    - ❑ Arts or technology education
    - ❑ Travel or transitions
    - ❑ Small group or special classroom
    - ❑ Bathroom
    - ❑ Physical education or sports
    - ❑ Vocational settings
    - ❑ Extracurricular or co-curricular

2. In which of the environments listed above is the child unable or unwilling to participate in the tasks and activities expected of all students despite the accommodations or assistance provided?

    _____
    _____

3. Within the above environments, specify where the child needs additional or specialized strategies or accommodations to adequately participate in these general tasks or activities:

Activity	*Environment*
Safety	_____
Maintaining or changing positions	_____
Maintaining cleanliness or hygiene	_____
Eating or drinking	_____
Traveling	_____
Managing clothing	_____
Using tools, materials, or toys	_____
Storing materials, setup, cleanup	_____
Beginning or completing tasks	_____
Recording information	_____
Moving in play or leisure activities	_____
Communicating	_____
Interacting in a positive way	_____
Regulating own behavior	_____
Following rules and adult direction	_____
Understanding or remembering	_____

4. I tried these strategies for helping the child meet specific expectations:

Strategy	*Expectation*
_____	_____
_____	_____
_____	_____
_____	_____
_____	_____

5. I feel an occupational therapist could provide additional strategies to help the child meet the following expectations in school:

    _____
    _____
    _____
    _____
    _____

(Adapted from AOTA, 1994; BCHCEB, 1993; W. J. Coster, 1996; and R. O. Smith, 1993.)

Figure 7 Sample Reference Guide for Teachers: Physical Therapy

1. What are the environments in which I frequently observe the child? *Check ALL that apply.*
   - ❑ General classroom, large groups
   - ❑ Cafeteria or snack area
   - ❑ Recess or playground
   - ❑ Arts or technology education
   - ❑ Travel or transitions
   - ❑ Small group or special classroom
   - ❑ Bathroom
   - ❑ Physical education or sports
   - ❑ Vocational settings
   - ❑ Extracurricular or co-curricular

2. The child shows problems moving in the environments listed above, despite the accommodations or assistance I have provided:

   _____

   _____

3. Within the above environments, the child demonstrates difficulty with posture or movement in these activities.

Activity	*Environment*
Walking	
Managing stairs, ramps, curbs, changes in terrain	_____
Maintaining a sitting or standing position	_____
Changing positions	
Keeping up with peers (tires easily, low endurance)	_____
Getting from one place to the next without getting lost	_____
Using playground or gym equipment	_____
Maneuvering a wheelchair	_____
Managing transfers	_____
Opening doors, lockers	_____
Toileting	_____
Other	_____

4. I tried these strategies to help the child move safely:

Strategy	*Expectation*
_____	_____
_____	_____
_____	_____
_____	_____
_____	_____

5. I feel a physical therapist could provide additional strategies to help the child move more independently or safely in the following environments:

   _____

   _____

- enabling preschool children to participate in appropriate activities.

- establishing baseline data that corresponds to each annual goal and enables measurement of progress.

- teaching the child in the way he or she is most capable of learning.

The IEP team begins the evaluation process with the review of existing data to determine the need for additional tests. Existing data might include academic records, medical reports, previously administered standardized tests, and information gathered from parents and teachers. The IEP team may determine additional testing is needed. When conducting an evaluation, the IEP team uses more than one test or assessment tool, includes information from multiple sources, employs technically sound instruments, selects and administers tests that are free of bias towards the child's race or culture, and administers tests in the language or mode of communication most familiar to the child. Assessments and evaluation materials must be in the form most likely to yield accurate information about what the child knows and can do academically, developmentally, and functionally. Assessments or measures are valid and reliable for specific purposes. IEP teams should not use these materials for other purposes.

A standardized criterion-referenced test of functional skills, such as the School Function Assessment or School Assessment of Motor and Process Skills provides information specific to the child's functional performance and participation at school.

Standardized, norm-referenced tests sometimes serve the needs of OTs and PTs. However, an appropriate norm-referenced test may not be available or necessary and the therapist may choose a criterion-referenced test. A standardized criterion-referenced test of functional skills, such as the School Function Assessment (Coster, W. et al., 1998) or School Assessment of Motor and Process Skills (Fisher, A. G., et al., 2005) provides information specific to the child's functional performance and participation at school. At other times, no test exists that is valid for the child's age or disability, or the test's design yields information unrelated to the reason for the referral. Therapists may use non-standardized inventories to identify a child's actual performance in daily school routines and activities, and to determine what the student needs to do next. Therapists collect and report information in ways that are useful for establishing eligibility for special education and related services, as well as for program planning. No current law or practice requires OTs and PTs to obtain and report test scores as a means to determine eligibility for therapy services.

IDEA specifies that schools must educate children with disabilities in the least restrictive environment, with a preference for educating the child in the general education classroom. To support this process, OTs and PTs assess how the child functions in the context of the classroom, the cafeteria, the halls, the playground, the restroom, the bus, and anywhere else within the naturally occurring school environment.

Eligibility for Occupational Therapy and Physical Therapy

Before the IEP team discusses whether or not a student is eligible for occupational therapy or physical therapy, the IEP team determines if the student is a child with a disability. The definition of a child with a disability includes both impairment and a need for special education. First, the IEP team determines if the child meets the criteria for one of the impairment areas listed in Figure 1. Second, the team decides if the child needs special education. The IEP team considers evaluation data gathered by all members when making both decisions. The OT and PT share their professional judgments based on data gathered from the evaluation to help the team determine if the student is a child with a disability. If the IEP team includes an OT or PT and that team decides that the child has an impairment and needs special education, they can write an IEP at the meeting or schedule another IEP team meeting. The OT and PT help inform the team about the student's present level of academic achievement and functional performance as stated in the IEP, determine the child's educational needs, and develop goals that address those needs. The team then decides what kind of special education the child needs to meet the goals.

Next, the team asks the qualifying question for school occupational therapy and school physical therapy: is occupational therapy or physical therapy required to assist the child to benefit from special education? Being able to determine the need for these related services flows from knowing the nature of the special education the child will receive. The timing of this decision helps the team focus on the child's goals and the expertise needed to help meet them, rather than on identified deficits. Also, this timing moves the process away from using erroneous criteria to qualify or disqualify a child for occupational therapy or physical therapy. IEP teams should not use specific test scores, a percentage of developmental delay, or cognitive referencing for this purpose. Effgen states:

> "Under this concept, a child's potential for improvement in therapy is based on the relationship between intellectual and motor development. If a child's cognitive skills are lower than or equal to motor skills, then it is believed he would not benefit from physical therapy and would not be eligible for services. Studies have not supported cognitive referencing… Severe cognitive disability might limit or slow progress, but it should not be used in determining the need for or access to physical therapy. Recent research on those with severely limited physical and mental disabilities indicated that PT could be effective in helping those individuals achieve their goals, although generalization of skills was limited." (Effgen 2000, 125)

No one should assume that the therapist must address what he or she directly evaluated. Instead, occupational therapy and physical therapy evaluations contribute to the IEP team's understanding of the child's educational and functional needs. As team members, therapists participate in developing goals for the child and discussing strategies to help the child achieve the goals. The team decides if occupational therapy or physical therapy will be added to the IEP by applying IDEA's definition of related services: those that are "required to assist a child with a disability to benefit from special education."

The team asks the qualifying question for school occupational therapy and school physical therapy: is occupational therapy or physical therapy required to assist the child to benefit from special education?

Writing the IEP

The IEP is a systematic instructional planning tool, driven by a child's needs, that continues the work of the IEP team. It lays the groundwork for instruction. It is not a detailed instructional or intervention plan nor is it written by one person. The IEP refers to a document with specific components required by law; it also refers to the team's decision-making process that the law requires will move from referral to placement. The participants in the development of the IEP are a diverse group, each possessing knowledge and expertise that relate to the needs of the child, but working together for the benefit of that child. In doing so, this group fulfills the definition of collaborative consultation—an interactive process that enables people with diverse expertise to generate creative solutions to mutual problems. The nature of the process enhances and alters the group's outcomes, allowing them to produce solutions they could not have generated as individuals. (Idol, Paolucci-Whitcomb, and Nevin, 1987)

The IEP is a systematic instructional planning tool, driven by a child's unique needs.

Each participant plays an effective role. Parents know their child best, so they are a source of information and ideas for everyone involved. Teachers and therapists know how to develop successful experiences for the child in and beyond the classroom. Children must express their interests and have a clear understanding of their abilities as planning takes place. All these participants should

- come to the meeting prepared, on time, and organized.

- respect confidentiality.

- display empathy and positive regard toward the other participants.

- use non-judgmental statements.

- make a concerted effort to write the IEP collaboratively.

- continually evaluate the appropriateness of the program and pursue ongoing consultation activities with other participants.

Each participant in the IEP team meeting should come with some notes or ideas he or she would like the group to incorporate into the child's goals. Some districts start with a blank flip chart, white board, or projected computer page and as the discussion unfolds, the team writes the IEP. Or, staff may bring a draft IEP to the meeting but must be ready to make changes and revisions. In developing each child's IEP, the IEP team must consider

- the strengths of the child.

- the concerns of the parents for enhancing the education of their child.

- the results of the initial or most recent evaluation of the child.

- the academic, developmental, and functional needs of the child. (CFR 300.324)

Components of the IEP

Present Level of Academic Achievement and Functional Performance

The present level of academic achievement and functional performance is a narrative statement written in objective, measurable terms that answers the key question: *What is the child doing now?* The OT and PT add to the discussion about the child's functional performance. Occupational therapy and physical therapy evaluations provide valuable information about functional activities and tasks the student can perform, as well as the student's current level of participation in classroom and school activities. This present level should contain measurable baseline data for goals. Information from the occupational therapy and physical therapy evaluations helps establish a baseline from which the team develops goals and measures progress.

Standards-based IEPs link academic standards to the IEP team's discussion of the present level of academic achievement and functional performance, as well as to annual goals. Knowing and understanding the academic standards and expectations for all students at a specific grade or age level allows the IEP team to accurately appraise the student's learning needs. This results in goals that are reasonable, relevant, achievable, individualized and designed to ensure progress and involvement in the general education curriculum. Standards-based IEPs set annual goals for academic content areas based on the student's disability-related needs in reference to the academic standards, local curriculum and expectations for peers. By using standards-based IEPs, the team avoids focusing only on the student's individual skills and merely identifying the next skill to be mastered. (Wisconsin Department of Public Instruction, 2009, 5)

Annual Goals

After establishing present level of academic achievement and functional performance, the IEP team develops the student's measurable annual academic and functional goals. Annual goals are linked to a child's present level of academic achievement and functional performance and describe a reasonable expectation of the child's achievement within one year in priority areas. As such, the IEP team should write goals specifically enough so that anyone working with the child could determine if he or she has achieved that goal. Broad statements such as *improve fine motor skills* or *improve gross motor skills* do not describe a year's achievement that is readily recognizable. In contrast, one can objectively measure an annual goal like *complete all writing assignments independently* or *travel to and within all classrooms and common areas independently*. The team should also avoid using a test score or age equivalency to describe a level of attainment. Achievement linked to a particular test or developmental age is likely to be less understandable to the child's parent and may not reflect what the child needs to do in the school environment during the coming year.

Annual goals are designed so the child can be involved and make progress within the general education curriculum. For the preschool child, the goals describe the child's involvement in age-appropriate activities. The IEP team

Annual goals are linked to a child's present level of academic achievement and functional performance and describe a reasonable expectation of the child's achievement within one year.

collaboratively answers the key question: *What should the child be doing?* Goals typically consist of three parts:

- Functional behavior (what the child will do)

- Context (where or when)

- Criteria (to what measurable level and consistency)

IDEA no longer requires that annual goals include short-term objectives or benchmarks except for students who will take alternate assessments. Districts may choose to include short-term objectives or benchmarks in students' IEP goals. Short-term objectives (STO) are sequential or parallel milestones toward the achievement of an annual goal. They identify a logical breakdown of at least two major components between the present level and the annual goal. An STO is composed of a specific description of an observable behavior that one can measure and record. If the IEP participants do not expect a child to achieve independence in a skill within a year, they may write objectives that describe the goal with terms like, an *ability to tolerate, cooperate with, direct, or assist with* an activity. Benchmarks provide a schedule or timeframe for meeting milestones toward achieving the goal.

The IEP should not include a separate page of occupational therapy goals and a separate page of physical therapy goals. The IEP team as a whole writes the child's goals for academic and functional performance. The goals describe activities and behaviors that the child will demonstrate in the classroom and other educational environments, and are not discipline-specific. Tools that may assist the IEP team in writing the child's goals are the *School Function Assessment* (Coster et al., 1998) for students in kindergarten through sixth grade, and the *Enderle-Severson Transition Rating Scale* (Enderle and Severson, 2003) for older students.

IEP goals describe activities and behaviors that the child will demonstrate in the classroom and other educational environments, and are not discipline-specific.

Using the *School Function Assessment*, the IEP team could write the following goal: *The student will travel independently throughout the school building.* This goal is not discipline specific. It may require the OT to orient the student to the building. The PT may work with the student on balance so the student can move on slippery surfaces. The PT also may collaborate with the classroom teacher to help the teacher cue the student to walk with crutches in the classroom and hallways.

Using the *Enderle-Severson Transition Rating Scale*, the IEP team could write the following goal: *The learner independently gets from home or school to community resources (i.e., bank, library, clinic, post office, laundromat, and restaurant).* The goal is not discipline specific. It may require the teacher to instruct the student to read a map, find a bus route, or call a taxi for a ride. The PT may work with the student on strengthening exercises to enable the student to manage curbs and bus steps. The OT may work with the student to use visual cues to signal the bus at the desired stop and cross the street safely.

IEP goals should be functional, clear, jargon free, and address necessary skills. The *Goal Functionality Scale II* (McWilliam 2005) in Figure 8 on page 34 is a tool to help staff assess written IEP goals for these characteristics. Examples of goals that occupational therapy or physical therapy may collaborate to support are in Figure 9, which appears on pages 39.

Measuring and Reporting Progress

The IEP team decides how progress toward meeting the annual goals will be measured and when parents will be informed of their child's progress. The OT and PT discuss this during the IEP meeting. They also contribute information on how much progress the student shows in meeting IEP goals when the progress report is sent to parents. There is no requirement in law for each service provider on the IEP to send a progress report to parents. Since therapists, educators and parents all agree that ongoing, two-way communication supports positive student outcomes, the greater the number of service providers involved in progress reports, the more likely parents will understand services as a whole.

IEP teams sometimes ask questions about using standardized tests to measure progress toward annual goals. These instruments do not collect pre- and post-intervention data, and repeated use is not the purpose for which they are designed. Such instruments are standardized for point-in-time diagnostic testing. With repeated or frequent use the child may learn the test, or the test may assess a stable characteristic of the child that requires accommodation rather than remediation. It is more accurate and useful to the child for therapists and teachers to identify specific functional behaviors that they can see or hear and count in a naturally occurring context. There are various ways to measure progress on annual goals, some of which include teacher and therapist data in the form of charting, child work samples, data from observations of the child performing the targeted skill, informal pre- and post-testing data, and anecdotal records. Chapter 4 provides more detail on selected methods of counting behavior and progress monitoring.

Baseline data in the student's present level of academic achievement and functional performance as well as measurable goals in the IEP makes documentation of progress easier.

Having baseline data in the student's present level of academic achievement and functional performance as well as measurable goals in the IEP makes documentation of progress easier. The child's present level will quantify specific functional behaviors, such as how often the child performs a skill, under what conditions the skill is performed, or the fluency of the skill. The annual goal statement, including any objectives, will describe the same skill in the same quantified way. Periodic measures of progress indicate if the child is moving toward the goal and at what rate. It is more understandable to everyone involved to state the specific measurable behavior or skill directly in the IEP, along with the baseline measurement and goal measurement, rather than referring to an external standard like a test score.

Figure 8 Goal Functionality Scale II

Child Name or ID		Functional Domains E = engagement	
Goal/Outcome #		I = independence SR = social relationships	
Rater's Initials			

1. Is this skill GENERALLY USEFUL (i.e., can you answer *why* and *who cares;* broad enough yet specific enough)? If YES,			5	
2. ...If NOT REALLY USEFUL,			4	
3. ...If NOT AT ALL USEFUL,			3	
4. During duration of interaction with people or objects sustains attention (E)	+1	12. Cannot tell in what normalized contexts it would be useful	-1	
5. Persistence (E)	+1	13. Purpose is not evident or useful	-1	
6. Developmentally and contextually appropriate construction (E)	+1	14. Some element makes little sense	-1	
7. Pragmatic communication (SR)	+1	15. Unnecessary skill	-1	
8. Naturalistic social interaction (SR)	+1	16. Jargon	-1	
9. Friendship (SR)	+1	17. Increase/decrease	-1	
10. Developmentally appropriate independence in routines (not just a reflection of prompt level) (I)	+1	18. Vague	-1	
		19. Insufficient criterion	-1	
11. Participation in developmentally appropriate activities (E)	+1	20. Criterion present but does not reflect a useful level of behavior	-1	
SCORE				

This scale is designed to rate one IEP objective at a time. Because IEP goals are often statements about the domain addressed (e.g., Johnny will improve in communication), they barely serve as behavioral goals. The appropriate behavioral goal therefore is the more specific short-term objective, sometimes known as benchmark.

1. Complete the three top-left boxes. Assign a number to each outcome/objective.
2. Items 1-3: Read the outcome/objective and circle the appropriate usefulness score (i.e., 5, 4, or 3).
3. Items 4-11: Circle the scores matching the content of the outcome/objective. Note that the codes for these pertain to the three functional domains listed in the top right box.
4. Items 12-20: Circle the scores matching the flaws in the outcome/objective.
5. Score: Beginning with the general usefulness score, add 1 for each +1 circled and subtract 1 for each -1 circled. Enter the resulting score in the score box. This score could be a negative integer (e.g., -2). A high score in the positive range indicates greater goal functionality.

R. A. McWilliam. 2005. Vanderbilt Center for Child Development. Reprinted with permission.

Services

An IEP must include a statement of the special education, related services, supplementary aids and services, and program modifications and supports for school personnel that the school district will provide to enable the child to

- advance appropriately toward attaining the annual goals.

- be involved in and make progress in the general education curriculum.

- participate in extracurricular and other nonacademic activities.

- be educated and participate with other children with and without disabilities.

Special Education

Special education is a service that every child with an IEP will receive. The IEP team that affirmed a child's need for special education during the determination of eligibility will revisit the need for special education after writing the child's annual goals. The IEP team members will identify the specific special education that will be provided to help the child reach the annual goals. One simple example of special education is supplementary instruction in reading.

Related Services

IDEA defines related service as "transportation, and such developmental, corrective and other supportive services (including speech language pathology and audiology services, psychological services, physical and occupational therapy…) as may be required to assist a child with a disability to benefit from special education." The IEP team that includes an OT or PT decides whether the child needs occupational therapy or physical therapy, respectively, to benefit from special education. This decision is facilitated if the OT and PT use a functional assessment, such as the *School Function Assessment,* in collaboration with other team members to share in the evaluation of the child. The results of this assessment help the IEP team identify areas of need that relate to the child's participation in actual school activities and environments. Earlier in this chapter, the section on *Eligibility for Occupational Therapy and Physical Therapy* described the process of determining the need for related services that Hanft and Place discuss in *The Consulting Therapist* (1996). Hanft and Place recommend that the IEP team waits until they write the child's annual goals and identify the specific special education that will be provided to help the child meet those goals, before determining whether the student needs occupational therapy or physical therapy. Hanft suggests asking,

1. What does the student need to learn?

2. Which strategies will facilitate the student's learning?

3. Whose expertise is needed to assist the student with achieving outcomes?

IDEA defines related service as services required to assist a child with a disability to benefit from special education.

Question three gives the IEP team options: either to state that the therapy evaluation contributed to determining eligibility, identifying present level, and formulating goals, but the specific services from the special education teacher are sufficient to help the child meet the goals. Conversely, the team may state that the therapist has unique knowledge and skills necessary for this child's goal achievement. This process focuses on the unique needs of the student in an educational environment rather than on identified deficits. Therapists are more certain of how their services relate to the special education and the projected educational outcomes. This process also helps IEP teams discontinue related services when parents or teachers are reluctant to let go of therapy but have no real rationale for continuing to provide it.

The process described above improves the likelihood of being able to decide if occupational therapy or physical therapy is required to assist the child to benefit from special education. Occupational therapy and physical therapy are related services. The criteria for occupational therapy and physical therapy are found in the definition of a related service: *Does the child need physical therapy to benefit from special education?* The IEP team cannot know the answer until the team decides what special education the child will receive.

Guiding questions such as those that follow about the performance demands of the educational environment and the child's ability to function within it will help the team integrate information from the occupational therapy evaluation and determine the need for service.

- Is the child having difficulty meeting high priority demands in educational environments of activities of daily living, assuming the student role, participating socially, playing, or pursuing leisure or vocational outcomes?

- What are the characteristics of the child, of the activities, and of the environment that promote or hinder success?

- Do the discrepancies between the child's performance and the demands of the activities or environment interfere with the child having equal opportunity to gain access to, benefit from, or participate in the educational program or services? For example, a child may need special education to learn mathematics, but limited eye-hand coordination may interfere with the use of manipulatives and with written expression of knowledge.

- Is intervention, collaboration with teachers, or mobilization of resources by the OT an effective and efficient way to improve the child's ability to function in the environment? In the example above, an OT may adapt the manipulatives and provide other assistive technology that allows the child to complete assignments.

The following guiding questions may assist the team in considering the PT's evaluation along with other staff reports to determine the child's need for physical therapy.

Does the child need occupational therapy or physical therapy to benefit from special education? The IEP team cannot know the answer until the team decides what special education the child will receive.

- Does the child have difficulty with functional mobility in classrooms, hallways, cafeteria, restroom, or playground which affects participation in school activities?

- Is the child able to negotiate stairs, ramps, inclines, exits, and slippery surfaces or travel safely throughout the outdoor campus?

- Is the child able to maintain or change positions in school settings to participate in educational activities and to manage self care?

- Is there potential for the child to participate in school activities with physical therapy intervention?

- Does the child have a progressive condition and therapy intervention is needed to prevent or alleviate functional limitations at school?

- Is the knowledge and expertise of the PT required to meet the child's needs or to collaborate with school personnel?

The OT or PT alone cannot answer these questions. Understanding one another's roles and skills and listening to each other's observations about the child will help the IEP team answer the questions together. Answering the questions may require any member of the team to relinquish former practices and domains in order to serve the child in the least restrictive environment.

Occupational therapy or physical therapy does not cure a child's medical condition, such as cerebral palsy, muscular dystrophy, or autism. Therapy helps the child with a disability perform important functions that support or enable participation in academic and nonacademic activities. When deciding whose expertise is needed to assist the child to meet IEP goals, IEP teams must recognize that according to the Wisconsin Physical Therapy Practice Act, only a PT or physical therapist assistant (PTA) under the supervision of a PT can provide physical therapy. The PT helps determine if the service is a physical therapy intervention that only the PT or the supervised PTA can provide or if this is a student activity that is part of classroom routines. Similarly, the OT helps determine if the service is an occupational therapy intervention that only the OT or the supervised occupational therapy assistant (OTA) can provide under state law.

Therapy helps the child with a disability perform important functions that support or enable participation in academic and nonacademic activities.

Supplementary Aids and Services
Supplementary aids and services are aids, services, and other supports that are provided in regular education classes, other education-related settings, and in extracurricular and nonacademic settings to enable a child with a disability to be educated with nondisabled children to the maximum extent appropriate. (CFR 300.42) The OT and PT participate in the IEP team discussion about the supplementary aids and services the student may need. The therapist helps the IEP team decide on assistive technology and adaptive devices for the student. The focus is upon adapting the environment or providing accommodations to allow student participation in school routines. The amount, frequency, duration and location of supplementary aids and services are documented on the student's

IEP. Typically, the condition or specific circumstances when the equipment will be used are written in this section of the IEP. Figure 10 on page 40 provides examples of supplementary aids and services.

Program Modifications and Supports

Program modifications and supports for school personnel are services or activities that school personnel need in order to provide services. There is a relationship between supplementary aids and services for children and program modifications and supports for school personnel. For example, if a child needs assistance transferring from one chair to another (a supplementary service), a teacher or paraprofessional may need instruction from a PT on how to safely transfer the child (a support for school personnel). The OT and PT participate in the IEP team discussion about the program modifications and supports for school personnel. When adaptive equipment will be used by personnel not licensed as an OT, OTA, PT, or PTA, the IEP team documents the specific equipment, training by the therapist in the use of the equipment, provision of safety guidelines and usage log in the IEP. They also document the amount, frequency, duration, and location in the IEP. Appendix E provides sample forms for recording information about adaptive equipment. Examples of program modifications and supports for school personnel are in Figure 11on page 41.

Amount of Service

The IEP team decides on the amount, frequency, duration and location of services the student will receive in order to attain the annual goal. The OT and PT participate in this determination. The preferred practice patterns in the *Guide to Physical Therapist Practice* offer some direction in the amount of physical therapy in terms of expected number of visits per episode of care. (American Physical Therapy Association, 1999, Ch 4–7) Some requirements for documenting amount, frequency, location and duration of services are listed below.

- The amount of therapy must be stated in the IEP so that the level of the agency's commitment of resources is clear to parents and all who are involved in the IEP development and implementation.

- The amount of therapy may be stated as a range. A range may be used for specific circumstances or conditions based on the unique needs of the child. A range may not be based on staff availability or schedules.

- The amount of time per episode/session/day/week must be appropriate to the service.

- The amount of therapy should be based upon the student's needs, not the availability of staff.

- The duration of service is considered the length of the IEP unless otherwise stated. When the duration is different than the rest of the IEP, the IEP should show beginning and ending dates.

When adaptive equipment will be used, the IEP team documents the specific equipment, training by the therapist in the use of the equipment, provision of safety guidelines and usage log in the IEP.

Figure 9 Examples of Goals and Objectives

Present level of functional performance: Kaitlin walks independently in classrooms and bathrooms with a reverse walker. She obtained a motorized wheelchair which she will learn to use for longer distances.	
Annual goal: Kaitlin will travel independently throughout the school environment using her reverse walker and motorized wheelchair by meeting the following objectives:	

Short-term objectives	Comments
Kaitlin will independently move from chair, toilet, or floor to motorized wheelchair using the reverse walker. Kaitlin will independently maneuver motorized wheelchair from one classroom to another. Kaitlin will move through hallways and cafeteria lines in her motorized wheelchair without bumping into others. Kaitlin will independently exit the building and move safely around areas surrounding the school in her motorized wheelchair.	The skill is important as Kaitlin will participate in daily school routines and activities. The settings are clearly stated and the criterion (independence) represents a functional level of behavior. The objectives address acquisition and generalization from classroom to outside the school building. Independent travel allows for naturalistic social interactions with peers.

Present level of functional performance: Using the positioning system or customized wheelchair, Jason maintains posture for at least 20 minutes during classroom instruction.	
Annual goal: Using the positioning system or customized wheelchair in the classroom, Jason will type 100 words in 35 minutes with the headpointer switch.	

Benchmarks	Comments
By December 1, Jason will type 50 words in 25 minutes with the headpointer switch in the classroom. By April 4, Jason will type 80 words in 30 minutes with the headpointer switch in the classroom.	The goal and benchmarks are useful in allowing Jason to be involved in the curriculum. The classroom context is clear and the criterion is set in the benchmarks and specified times for the behavior to occur. Time in the classroom allows for naturalistic social interactions with peers.

Annual goal: While playing with at least one other student, Ed will share and interact with toys without banging or throwing them without adult assistance five times per day for 10 minutes.

Comments: This social-emotional goal is an age appropriate activity for a four year old child. The condition is clearly stated and the criterion is included in the annual goal statement without the use of objectives or benchmarks. It describes a behavior that is specific, measurable and functional for the child, without specifying the services that will support his achievement of the outcome.

Figure 10 Examples of Supplementary Aids and Services

Supplementary aids and services: aids, services, and other supports provided to or on behalf of the student in regular education or other educational settings. Yes ☑ No ☐ (If yes, describe below)	Frequency/Amount	Location	Duration
Sit in 12" chair with arms and wedge cushion	Whenever child participates in fine motor activities at the 24" table with peers	Special education and regular classroom	Same as IEP dates
Stand in the Easy Stander	When chemistry lab assignment requires work at the lab counter	Regular classroom	Same as IEP dates
No limitation on student moving, standing, or pacing in the back of the classroom	Whenever a test or assignment is longer than 5 questions, until student completes the test or assignment.	Regular classroom	Same as IEP dates

Figure 11 Examples of Program Modifications and Supports

Program modifications or supports for school personnel that will be provided. Yes ☑ No ☐ (If yes, describe below)	Frequency/ Amount	Location	Duration
Consultation among special education teacher, general education teacher, OT and PT	30 minutes each time, twice per semester	General education classroom	Same as IEP dates
OT will provide training for teacher and classroom aide on positioning Carlos in chair at table	3 sessions, 20 minutes each	General education classroom	September 7, (year) to October 15, (year)
PT will provide training for teacher and classroom aide on lifting techniques	5 sessions, thirty minutes each	General education classroom	September 7, (year) to November 7, (year)

Figure 12 Examples of Amount, Frequency and Location

- Typical: Direct occupational therapy two times per week for 30-minute sessions in the regular classroom.
- Short-Term Intensive: Direct physical therapy five times per week at 45 minutes each session for the first semester outside the regular classroom.
- Infrequent: Occupational therapy four times during the second semester, for 25 minutes each session.
- Group: Physical therapy for one hour, two times per week, in a group of three children in the regular classroom.
- Conditional: When the child does not get to class on time on two consecutive days, occupational therapy will be provided for 6-8 sessions of 30 minutes each outside the regular classroom.
- Predicted Schedule:

  September 1 – November 1   Physical therapy three times per week 40 minutes per session outside the regular classroom.

  November 2 – January 15   Physical therapy two times per week, 30 minutes per session in the regular classroom.

  January 16 – June 3   Physical therapy 30 minutes once per week in the regular classroom.

- Location designates whether the student receives services in the regular class or outside the regular class. *Regular class* means with nondisabled peers. Services provided outside the regular class are considered removal from regular education.

Figure 12 on the previous page provides examples of amount, frequency and location. DPI Information Update Bulletin 10.07 (Wisconsin DPI 2010c) provides more guidance and specific examples on how to describe the amount of special education, related services, supplementary aids and services, and program modifications and support for school personnel in students' IEPs.

Least Restrictive Environment

Both federal and state laws require that, to the maximum extent appropriate, school districts educate children with disabilities with children who do not have disabilities. The team that develops the child's IEP determines the least restrictive environment (LRE) for the implementation of the child's IEP from a continuum of locations and service options. They identify the environment in which a child will receive special education and related services. The discussion begins with the ideal: consideration of services in the student's neighborhood school, in the regular classroom with nondisabled peers. The IEP team determines the extent to which a child will not participate in the regular education environment and documents those determinations on the IEP. They may remove a child from the regular educational environment only when teachers cannot educate the child satisfactorily in the regular classroom using supplementary aids and services, due to the nature or severity of the child's disability. The team must determine the child's placement annually and base the selection on the child's IEP and on specific requirements in the law. The team may not select an environment based solely on

The team discussion begins with the ideal: consideration of services in the student's neighborhood school, in the regular classroom with nondisabled peers.

- the category of the child's disability.

- the availability of related services.

- curriculum or space.

- school policy.

- administrative convenience.

- the configuration of the delivery system.

- perceived attitudes of regular education staff or children.

LRE pertains to school-based therapy as well as the educational services that teachers provide. Some children require individual intervention that the therapist cannot provide in a classroom. The nature of the intervention, the space or equipment required in the therapy, or the potential distraction to other children are acceptable reasons for the therapist to implement the child's IEP in a location other than a classroom full of other children. In most instances, however, the actual classroom, playground, gym or other natural environment is the LRE. The IEP team documents the location(s) for occupational therapy and physical therapy and describes them in terms of the extent to which the child will be removed from education with nondisabled peers.

Delivery of occupational therapy and physical therapy within the least restrictive environment is consistent with the collaborative model of service delivery. Collaboration among team members can result in reduced duplication of services, more consistent attention to the child's needs throughout the school day, and more relevant application of the knowledge and skills of individual disciplines to educational difficulties that children experience. Teachers and therapists now recognize that they cannot ensure educational relevance through isolated, pull-out services. To promote educational relevance, OTs and PTs must observe and work with children in the context of educational programs, whether services are direct or indirect. (Rainforth, B. and York-Barr, 1997) For many school teams, this requires a considerable change in roles and practices.

To provide services for preschoolers in the LRE means serving children in natural environments and age-appropriate settings with typically developing peers. This may mean serving children at home or in daycare, Head Start, or private preschool. The IEP team considers the child's educational, behavioral, and social needs. Presently, 98 percent of children in Birth to 3 programs are served in natural environments. There is an expectation these children will be served in natural environments when they make the transition to public school programs. The National Individualizing Preschool Inclusion Project comprises three components that apply to preschool occupational therapy and physical therapy. (McWilliam and Clingenpeel 2005)

- Functional intervention planning is carried out principally through a routines-based assessment, featuring an interview of the family and the teaching staff.

- Integrated therapy consists of specialists using models labeled individualized within routines and group activity to provide special education and related services.

- Embedded intervention involves the use of proven instructional principles, especially incidental teaching, in the context of developmentally appropriate activities. For example, embedded interventions allow practice of motor skills within classroom and school activities.

OTs and PTs frequently follow an itinerant model of serving preschool children with disabilities. In the itinerant model, the therapist delivers IEP services or consults with personnel to implement the IEP in regular education settings in the community or school district. For instance, in the community, a child might receive services in the child's home, a state-licensed child care center, a Head Start setting, a school-sponsored play group, a YMCA program, or a public library program. In a school district, a child might receive services in a four-year-old kindergarten or Title I preschool program. Using the IEP for guidance the itinerant therapist not only works directly with the child but also

To promote educational relevance, OTs and PTs must observe and work with children in the context of educational programs, whether services are direct or indirect.

collaborates with the child care teacher and other service providers in the development of activities and educational objectives. In this model, the therapist focuses on the needs of the target child without *pulling the child out* of the environment that the IEP team determined was least restrictive for the child. Detailed information about serving preschool children in the LRE is in *DPI Information Update Bulletin 10.03: Free Appropriate Public Education (FAPE) in the Least Restrictive Environment (LRE) for Preschoolers (age 3-5) with Disabilities.* (Wisconsin DPI 2010b)

Re-evaluation

The IEP team conducts a reevaluation of a child who has a current IEP if the educational or related services needs of the child, including improved academic achievement and functional performance, warrant a reevaluation; or if the child's parent or teacher requests a reevaluation. (34 CFR 300.303(a) A reevaluation occurs at least every three years and not more than once a year, unless agreed otherwise by parent and the district. A reevaluation always begins with review of existing information. When a student's IEP includes occupational therapy and physical therapy, therapists participate in the reevaluation process.

Adding to a Student's Existing IEP

Adding occupational therapy or physical therapy to a student's existing IEP requires a reevaluation.

Since IDEA 1997 and again since IDEA 2004, DPI has advised that adding occupational therapy or physical therapy to a student's existing IEP requires a reevaluation. OTs and PTs are regulated not only by special education law, but also by state professional practice acts, those requirements that regulate a therapist's professional practice and licensing standards. Practice act requirements and licensing standards apply to occupational therapy and physical therapy in all settings, including school-based practice. This includes evaluating a child before providing services. So, if a district is considering occupational therapy or physical therapy for a current IEP, it must initiate a reevaluation process that includes a notice to the parent of reevaluation, review of existing information by the IEP team with a decision about the need for additional testing, and consent from the parent for testing. Occupational therapy and physical therapy are unique in this respect; other services can be added at an IEP team meeting without conducting a reevaluation. The review of existing information is likely to negate the need for parallel testing by other IEP team members and make the process simpler. The next three-year reevaluation date changes, but a reevaluation always can be conducted sooner if needed.

Discontinuing Occupational Therapy or Physical Therapy

Occupational therapy and physical therapy can be removed from the IEP at an annual IEP team meeting or any other IEP team meeting. The criterion for including or not including occupational therapy and physical therapy on a child's IEP is whether or not the child with a disability requires the related service to benefit from special education. School districts should not develop any other criteria or guidelines. The IEP team comes to consensus on this decision in the same way that they determined the initial need for the respective therapy. They review or revise the child's annual goals and identify the specific special education that will be provided to help the child meet those goals. Dismissal occurs when the IEP team decides that the child no longer requires therapy to benefit from special education. For example, when a child reaches an IEP goal that the therapist supported, or the therapist's knowledge, skill, or expertise is no longer needed to help the student reach the goal, the new IEP will not include the related service.

Using measurable data gives the therapist, parent, and other IEP team members objective information on which to base their decision. The child's present level of academic achievement and functional performance should provide measurable baseline data. The IEP goals describe the same behavior in a measurable way. By periodically collecting data and making comparisons to baseline data, the IEP team can determine progress toward accomplishing the IEP goal. This process is not considered an IEP team evaluation or reevaluation, so parental consent is not required.

Parents may be fearful that a discontinued service will never be offered to their child again. It is helpful to reassure the parent that the IEP team will reconsider occupational therapy and physical therapy based upon new needs or challenges that the child may have, such as transition from elementary school to middle school or preparing for transition from high school to adult life.

There are other ways in which an IEP team may discontinue a child's occupational therapy or physical therapy. The team may write beginning and ending dates as the duration of the service on the child's IEP. When the ending date is reached, the therapy will end without another IEP team meeting. The therapy will not be included in the next annual IEP team meeting or three-year reevaluation unless the need for it is suspected. A second way is through a reevaluation, when the team finds that the child no longer needs any special education. Without special education, the child will not have an IEP or any related services. A third way occurs when a parent of a child with a disability or an adult student revokes consent for special education and related services. The parents of a child who receives an initial evaluation as a child with a disability will be asked to give informed consent in writing for the child to receive special education services, before any services begin. The parent has the right to consent or refuse to consent. The parent or the student, if an adult, also may revoke consent for services at any time after the special education has begun. Revocation of consent applies to all IEP services. A parent cannot choose to revoke consent for some services and keep others. For example, a parent cannot revoke consent for speech and language services and keep physical therapy. The revocation of consent must be in writing. Upon receipt of the written revocation, the school district promptly provides prior written notice before stopping special education and related services. The school district may not use mediation or due process procedures to challenge the parent's revocation of consent. Once special education and related services end, the school district is not required to make a free and appropriate public education (FAPE) available to the child and is not

Dismissal occurs when the IEP team decides that the child no longer requires therapy to benefit from special education.

required to have an IEP team meeting or develop an IEP for the child. The school district also is not required to offer the child discipline protections under IDEA. The school district is not required to amend the child's education records to remove any reference to the child's receipt of special education and related services. However, if the child is referred for special education in the future, the district must act upon that referral, and the evaluation will be treated as an initial evaluation.

Extended School Year Services

Special education and related services provided beyond the limits of the school term and documented on an IEP are Extended School Year (ESY) services. A child's IEP team must consider, as appropriate, whether a child needs ESY services in order to receive a FAPE. The district is not required to consider ESY services for each child at an IEP meeting. The child's IEP team makes the determination of whether or not ESY services will be included on the IEP. ESY services typically occur over the summer break, but can occur any time that school is not in session. Occupational therapy or physical therapy may be the only service provided during ESY.

Federal special education regulations and court cases establish a standard for determining whether a child is eligible for ESY services. In most cases, courts consider a child's regression during an interruption in services and the child's recoupment of skills after services resume in determining eligibility for ESY services. Some other factors that the IEP team may consider include but are not limited to the

Special education regulations and court cases establish a standard for ESY services, including regression during an interruption in services and the child's recoupment of skills after services resume.

- degree of impairment.

- ability of the child's parents to provide the educational structure at home.

- child's rate of progress.

- child's behavioral and physical problems.

- availability of alternative resources.

- ability of the child to interact with children without disabilities.

- areas of the child's curriculum which need continuous attention.

- child's vocational needs.

- whether the requested service is extraordinary for the child's condition, as opposed to an integral part of a program for those with the child's condition.

An extensive description of ESY and frequently asked questions are in *DPI Information Update 10.02, Extended School Year.* (Wisconsin DPI 2010a)

References

34 CFR Parts 300 and 301, IDEA Final Regulations. http://idea.ed.gov/download/finalregulations.pdf (accessed June 25, 2010) .

American Physical Therapy Association. 1999. *Guide to Physical Therapist Practice*. Alexandria, VA: American Physical Therapy Association.

Brown County Children with Disabilities Educational Board, 1993. *Occupational/Physical Therapy Teacher Questionnaire*. Green Bay, Wisconsin.

Coster, W. 1996. *Overview of the School Function Assessment*. Presented at the annual conference of the American Occupational Therapy Association, Chicago, IL, April 22, 1996.

Coster, W., T. Deeney, J. Haltiwanger, and S. Haley. 1998. *School Function Assessment*. San Antonio, Texas: Therapy Skill Builders a division of the Psychological Corporation.

Effgen, S. 2000. "Factors Affecting the Termination of Physical Therapy Services for Children in School Settings." *Pediatric Physical Therapy* 12(3): 121–26.

Enderle, J. and S. Severson. 2003. Enderle-Severson Transition Rating Scale, Third Edition. Moorhead, MN.

Fisher, A., K. Bryze, V. Hume, and L. A. Griswold. 2005. *School AMPS: School Version of the Assessment of Motor and Process Skills*. Fort Collins, CO: Three Star Press.

Hanft, B. and P. Place. 1996. *The Consulting Therapist: A Guide for OTs and PTs in Schools*. San Antonio: Pearson Education, Inc.

Idol, L., P. Paolucci-Whitcomb, and A. Nevin. 1987. *Collaborative Consultation*. Austin, TX. PRO-ED.

McWilliam, R. 2005. Goal Functionality Scale II. The National Individualizing Preschool Inclusion Project, a "Project of National Significance" funded by the U.S. Department of Education, Office of Special Education Programs.

McWilliam, R. and B. Clingenpeel. "What is the Individualizing Inclusion Model?" National Individualizing Preschool Inclusion Project. Presented at the Statewide School Therapy Conference, Wisconsin Dells, WI, October 28, 2005.

Rainforth, B. and J. York-Barr. 1997. *Collaborative Teams for Students with Severe Disabilities,* 2nd Edition. Baltimore: Paul H. Brookes Publishing Co., Inc.

Smith, R.O. 1993. "Technology Part II: Adaptive Equipment and Technology." In *Classroom Applications for School-Based Practice*. Ed. C.B. Royeen. Rockville, MD: American Occupational Therapy Association.

Wisconsin Department of Public Instruction. 2009. A *Guide to Connecting Academic Standards and IEPs.* http://www.dpi.wi.gov/sped/pdf/iepstandardsguide.pdf (accessed March 23, 2010).

___. 2010a. DPI *Information Update Bulletin 10.02: Extended School Year.* http://dpi.wi.gov/sped/bul10-02.html (accessed September 10, 2010).

___. 2010b. *DPI Information Update Bulletin 10.03: Free Appropriate Public Education (FAPE) in the Least Restrictive Environment (LRE) for Preschoolers (age 3-5) with Disabilities.* http://dpi.wi.gov/sped/bul10-03.html (accessed September 10, 2010).

___. 2010c. *DPI Information Update Bulletin 10.07: Describing Special Education, Related Services, Supplementary Aids and Services, and Program Modifications and Supports.* http://dpi.wi.gov/sped/bul10-07.html (accessed November 15, 2010).

Other Resources

Chiarello, L. and S. Effgen. 2006. "Updated Competencies for Physical Therapists Working in Early Intervention." *Pediatric Physical Therapy* 18(2): 148–58.

Cole, K., P. Mills, and S. Harris. 1991. "Retrospective Analysis of Physical and Occupational Therapy Progress in Young Children: An Examination of Cognitive Referencing." *Pediatric Physical Therapy* 3(4): 185-89.

"Collaborating Partners." http://www.collaboratingpartners.com/ (accessed July 21, 2010).

Wisconsin Department of Public Instruction. 2009. *A Guide for Writing IEPs.* http://www.dpi.wi.gov/sped/pdf/iepguide.pdf (accessed March 23, 2010)

School-Based Occupational Therapy

4

Occupational therapy means the therapeutic or constructive use of purposeful and meaningful occupations to evaluate and treat individuals of all ages who have a disease, disorder, impairment, activity limitation or participation restriction that interferes with their ability to function independently in daily life roles and environments and to promote health and wellness. (Chapter 448, Wis. Stats.) The word *occupation* in this specific context means engagement in activities of daily living, education, work, play, leisure and social participation. According to the American Occupational Therapy Association (AOTA), *occupation* encompasses intentional, action-oriented behavior that is personally meaningful. A person's unique characteristics and culturally based view of his or her roles determine this behavior. (AOTA 1995; Chapter 448, Wis. Stats.) When working with a child, the therapist, in collaboration with others, engages the child in activities that the child values or finds meaningful. If a child has not yet developed an understanding of his or her own purpose, the occupational therapist (OT) collaborates with the team to help the child explore activities that motivate and engage the child. The OT contributes to the design of such activities that will lead to functional performance patterns that are typical for children of the same age in similar environmental contexts. In school environments, these include academic and non-academic outcomes such as social skills, math, reading, writing, recess play, self-help skills, participation in sports, and preparation for post-high school education and employment.

OTs in schools evaluate children in the context of their educational environments, provide intervention, and communicate with educational personnel, parents, and community agencies and service providers.

OTs in schools evaluate children in the context of their educational environments, provide intervention including consultation services for and on behalf of children, and communicate with educational personnel, parents, and community agencies and service providers. Responsibilities of the OT in the school include

- participation in the IEP Team or 504 evaluations, either of which determines eligibility.

- participation in the development of the IEP or 504 plans, either of which determines goals and objectives for the child.

- development of an intervention plan to outline the specific occupational therapy intervention that will assist the child in meeting goals and objectives.

- provision of indirect and direct occupational therapy.

- reevaluation as indicated or required.

- provision of team support.

- provision of system support. (Hanft and Shepard 2008)

Conceptual Frameworks

There are two foundational systems, both of which have undergone significant revision, that OTs should know when practicing in Wisconsin schools: The *Occupational Therapy Practice Framework: Domain and Process* (herein called *Framework*) which AOTA adopted in 2002 and revised in 2008 as a means of outlining language and constructs that describe the profession's focus (AOTA 2002, AOTA 2008); and *Uniform Terminology for Occupational Therapy*, a system developed in 1979 and revised in 1989 and 1994. Professionals developed and revised these works at different points in the state's development of laws and standards. The *Framework* is used in professional literature and intervention planning, and *Uniform Terminology* is used in the Wisconsin Administrative Code, so it is helpful for the reader to become familiar with both systems. In addition, *The Guide to Occupational Therapy Practice* (Moyers and Dale, 2007) offers updates into professional understanding and awareness. A brief description of each system is provided in this chapter.

Two foundational systems that OTs should know when practicing in Wisconsin schools are The Occupational Therapy Practice Framework: Domain and Process, and Uniform Terminology for Occupational Therapy.

Occupational Therapy Practice Framework

The *Framework* describes both the domain and process of occupational therapy. As noted at the beginning of this chapter, the domain of occupational therapy is occupation in the broadest sense. Occupation is all of the things people do to occupy their time, many of which are day-to-day, routine activities. "Supporting health and participation in life through engagement in occupation" is the objective of occupational therapy intervention. (AOTA 2008) Figure 13 on the next page illustrates the aspects of occupational therapy domain. Figure 14 explains the aspects of each component of the domain.

Each of the terms used in Figures 13 and 14 are defined further in Figure 15 on page 53, and at length in the full *Framework* document. School OTs evaluate a child's ability to engage in age-appropriate areas of occupation. When engagement is inefficient or ineffective, the OT considers smaller units and sequences of performance known as performance skills and performance patterns. Performance skills and patterns are influenced by context and environment, demands of the activity, and client factors. In contrast to limited models of practice that view client factors and isolated performance skills as the sole targets of evaluation and intervention, the *Framework* recognizes the multiple, interrelated influences that determine a child's engagement in academic and functional activities. The components of occupational therapy domain as a whole thus drive the nature of the process of occupational therapy, including evaluation, intervention and outcome measurement. The *Framework* process will be compared to the IDEA process on page 56 in Figure 16.

Figure 13 Occupational Therapy Practice Framework: Domain

AOTA 2008. Reprinted with permission.

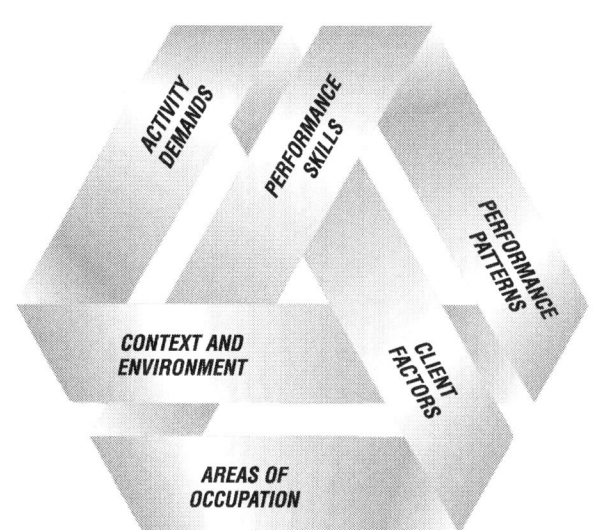

Figure 14 Occupational Therapy Practice Framework: Components of Domain AOTA 2008. Reprinted with permission.

Areas of Occupation	Client Factors	Performance Skills	Performance Patterns	Context and Environment	Activity Demands
Activities of Daily Living (ADL)*	Values, Beliefs, and Spirituality	Sensory Perceptual Skills	Habits	Cultural	Objects Used and their Properties
Rest and Sleep	Body Functions	Motor and Praxis Skills	Routines	Personal	
Education	Body Structures	Emotional Regulation Skills	Roles	Physical	Space Demands
Work			Rituals	Social	Social Demands
Play		Cognitive Skills		Temporal	
Leisure		Communication and Social Skills		Virtual	Sequencing and Timing
Social Participation					Required Actions
*Also referred to as *basic activities of daily living(BADL)* or *personal activities of daily living (PADL)*					Required Body Functions
					Required Body Structures

Uniform Terminology

The Wisconsin Administrative Code that governs the licensure and regulation of all OTs and occupational therapy assistants (OTAs) who practice in Wisconsin draws its terminology from the AOTA publication, *Uniform Terminology for Occupational Therapy-Third Edition* which predates the other relevant guides. (AOTA 1994) Chapter OT 1, Wis. Admin Code currently defines these terms:

> "Occupational performance areas" means the functional abilities that occupational therapy addresses in the areas of activities of daily living, including continence training; self maintenance; functional communication and functional mobility; work and productive activities, including home management; care giving; learning and vocational pursuits; and play or leisure activities, including solitary and social activities and recreation.

> "Occupational performance components" means the skills and abilities that an individual uses to engage in performance areas, including sensorimotor, sensory, neuromuscular and motor factors; cognitive integration and cognitive components; and psychological, social and self-management areas.

> "Occupational performance contexts" means situations or factors that influence an individual's engagement in desired or required occupational performance areas, including age, maturation, life cycle stage of disability, physical environment, social supports and expectations, and behavioral norms and opportunities. (Chapter OT 1.02, Wis. Admin Code)

These terms are slightly different and less comprehensive than the terms used in the *Framework*, but are comparable in concept. It is important for OTs and OTAs to understand and be able to use these terms accurately and effectively in their role documenting occupational therapy service in Wisconsin as described in Chapter OT 4.03(5)(b), Wis. Admin Code: "The individual's occupational performance areas and occupational performance components shall be routinely and systematically evaluated and documented."

Comparison of Terms

School OTs, school OTAs and other school staff will find it useful to compare the *Framework* used in professional literature, the *Uniform Terminology for Occupational Therapy* (UT-III) used in Wisconsin law, and the International Classification of Functioning, Disability and Health (ICF). The ICF is the World Health Organization's (WHO) document for the definition, measurement and policy formulations for health and disability worldwide. ICF integrates medical and social models of disability into one, holistic biopsychosocial model. In the medical model, disability is directly caused by disease, trauma or other health condition and requires medical treatment by professionals. "Disability, in this model, calls for medical or other treatment or intervention, to 'correct' the problem with the individual." (World Health Organization 2002) Conversely, the social model views disability as a socially created problem, not a problem within

The International Classification of Functioning, Disability and Health integrates medical and social models of disability into one, holistic biopsychosocial model.

Figure 15 Comparison of Terms (AOTA 2002. Reprinted with permission).

FRAMEWORK	UT-III	ICF
Occupations are "activities ... of everyday life, named, organized, and given value and meaning by individuals and a culture. Occupation is everything people do to occupy themselves, including looking after themselves, ... enjoying life ... and contributing to the social and economic fabric of their communities ... " (Law, Polatajko, Baptiste, & Townsend, 1997, p. 32).	Not addressed.	Not addressed.
Areas of occupation are various kinds of life activities in which people engage, including the following categories: Activities of daily living (ADL), instrumental activities of daily living (IADL), rest and sleep, education, work, play, leisure, and social participation.	**Performance areas-** • Activities of daily living • Work and productive activities • Play or leisure activities	**Activities and participation-** • **Activities-**"execution of a task or action by an individual" (p. 10). • **Participation-**"involvement in a life situation" (p.10). Examples of both: learning, task demands (routines), communication, mobility, self-care, domestic life, interpersonal interactions and relationships, major life areas, community, social and civic life. Activities and Participation from ICF overlap Areas of Occupation, Performance Skills, and Performance Patterns in the Framework.
Performance skills are features of what one does, not what one has, related to observable elements of action that have implicit functional purposes (adapted from Fisher & Kielhofner, 1995, p. 113). Performance skills include sensory perceptual, motor and praxis, emotional regulation, cognitive, communication and social skills.	**Performance components-**sensorimotor components, cognitive interaction and cognitive components, as well as psychosocial skills and psychological components. These components consist of some performance skills and some client factors as in the Framework (pp. 1052-1054).	**Activities and participation-** • **Activities-**"execution of a task or action by an individual" (p. 10). • **Participation-**"involvement in a life situation" (p.10). Examples of both: learning, task demands (routines), communication, mobility, self-care, domestic life, interpersonal interactions and relationships, major life areas, community, social and civic life. Activities and Participation from ICF overlap Areas of Occupation, Performance Skills, and Performance Patterns in the Framework.

FRAMEWORK	UT-III	ICF
Performance patterns are patterns of behavior related to daily life activities that occur with regularity. Performance patterns include habits, routines, roles and rituals.	Habits and routines are not addressed. Roles are listed as performance components (p. 1050).	**Activities and participation**- • **Activities**-"execution of a task or action by an individual" (p. 10). • **Participation**-"involvement in a life situation" (p.10). Examples of both: learning, task demands (routines), communication, mobility, self-care, domestic life, interpersonal interactions and relationships, major life areas, community, social and civic life. Activities and Participation from ICF overlap Areas of Occupation, Performance Skills, and Performance Patterns in the Framework.
Context and environment refers to a variety of interrelated conditions within and surrounding the client that influence performance. Context includes cultural, personal, physical, social, temporal, and virtual factors.	**Performance contexts** • **Temporal aspects** (chronological, developmental, life cycle, disability • **Environment** (physical, social, cultural)	**Contextual factors**-"represent the complete background of an individual's life and living. They include environmental factors and personal factors that may have an effect on the individual with a health condition and the individual's health and health-related states" (p. 16). • **Environmental factors**-"make up the physical, social and attitudinal environment in which people live and conduct their lives. The factors are external to individuals ... "(p. 16). • **Personal factors**-"the particular background of an individual's life and living ..." (p. 17) (e.g., gender, race, lifestyle, habits, social background, education, profession). Personal factors are not classified in ICF because they are not part of a health condition or health state, though they are recognized as having an effect on outcomes.
Activity demands are aspects of an activity, which include the objects used and their properties, space demands, social demands, sequencing and timing, required actions, required body functions and body structures needed to carry out the activity.	Not addressed.	Not addressed.

FRAMEWORK	UT-III	ICF
Client factors are those factors that reside within the client that may affect performance in areas of occupation. Client factors include • values, beliefs and spirituality • body functions • body structures	**Performance components**- sensorimotor components, cognitive interaction and cognitive components, as well as psychosocial skills and psychological components. These components consist of some performance skills and some client factors as presented in the Framework (pp. 1052-1054).	• **Body functions**-"the physiological functions of body systems (including psychological functions)" (p.10). • **Body structures**- "anatomical parts of the body such as organs, limbs and their components [that support body function]" (p. 10).

Note: FRAMEWORK = Occupational Therapy Practice Framework, Second Edition (AOTA 2008)
UT-III = Uniform Terminology for Occupational Therapy-Third Edition (AOTA 1994)
ICF = International Classification of Functioning (WHO 2001)

the individual. "In the social model, disability demands a political response, since the problem is created by an unaccommodating physical environment brought about by attitudes and other features of the social environment." The blending of these models in ICF reflects the view that disability and functioning are outcomes of interactions between challenges to health (diseases, disorders and injuries) and context. ICF emphasizes function, health, and participation rather than disease. (World Health Organization 2002) This model is compatible with the educational model described by IDEA, which emphasizes function, participation and academic achievement. Figure 15 on the previous page compares the terminology used in the *Framework*, Wisconsin law (UT-III) and the ICF. (AOTA 2002)

Occupational Therapy Initial Evaluation

Occupational therapy that is provided in public schools is governed by yet another conceptual framework: IDEA and state special education laws. In this context, occupational therapy is a potentially required related service to special education. When a parent, teacher or other individual believes that a child has a disability and needs special education, the individual makes a referral to the child's school for a special education evaluation. Referral is the first step in the special education process, followed by evaluation by an IEP team, as shown in Figure 2 in chapter 2. If there is any indication at the time of referral that the child might need occupational therapy, the IEP team must include an OT. (PI 11.24(2), Wis. Admin Code) State licensing and practice law also governs occupational therapy practice in schools. A therapist alone or in collaboration with an assistant must prepare an evaluation for each individual referred for services. (OT 4.03(3)(a), Wis. Admin Code) The resulting intervention for an individual child in school is always based on an occupational therapy evaluation that meets the standards of practice described in the state licensure law. The OT may use a variety of individual and collaborative processes to help the IEP team achieve the two purposes of an evaluation under IDEA: to determine if a child is a child with a disability, and to determine the educational needs of the child. (34 CFR, 300.301(c)(2))

If there is any indication at the time of referral that the child might need occupational therapy, the IEP team must include an OT.

Medical Referral and Medical Information

In Wisconsin, a school OT does not require a referral or prescription from a physician or other health care provider to conduct an initial evaluation as part of an IEP team, or to provide services for a child with a disability. Chapter OT 4.03(2)(e), Wis. Admin Code specifies,

> Physician order or referral from another health care provider is not required for evaluation or intervention if an OT or OTA provides services in an educational environment, including the child's home, for children and youth with disabilities pursuant to rules promulgated by the federal individuals with disabilities education act, the department of public instruction and the department of health and family services, or provides services in an educational environment for children and youth with disabilities pursuant to the code of federal regulations.

The exemption from a referral for occupational therapy in educational environments is specific to children or youth who have or are suspected to have a disability under IDEA, state special education law, or section 504 of the Rehabilitation Act.

A physician or other health care provider may send a referral or prescription for occupational therapy to the school or give it to the child's parent to share with the school. If the school district has not ever decided that the child has a disability, a school administrator should confirm the meaning of the referral: does the physician believe the child currently has a disability and requires a special education evaluation under Chapter 115.777, Wis. Stats? If the child already has been referred for a special education evaluation or has an IEP, the IEP team should consider the recommendation of the physician or other health care provider for occupational therapy. The IEP team, however, makes the final determination to provide occupational therapy to the child as a related service. The IEP team ultimately decides the necessary amount and frequency of the service, no matter what the physician recommends.

An OT must have medical information about a child before the child receives occupational therapy.

An OT must have medical information about a child before the child receives occupational therapy. (Chapter PI 11.24(9)(c) Wis. Admin Code) The therapist has a professional obligation to secure, review, and interpret the information that the parent, physician, or other health care professional provides. The therapist uses professional judgment to determine how much information is enough, and the amount may vary considerably from child to child. For example, when a child's medical condition is stable or uncomplicated, as is true of some children with learning disabilities, the therapist only may need to check periodically with the parents to see if new medical information is available. However, if the child is experiencing significant changes due to degenerative processes or surgical intervention, the therapist will require technical information from the physician.

Figure 16 Comparison of IEP Team Process with Occupational Therapy Process

Referral A teacher, parent, or other person refers the child for a special education evaluation.	**PI 11.24 (2)** IEP TEAM. If a child is suspected to need occupational therapy or physical therapy or both, the IEP team for that child shall include an appropriate therapist. (WI Admin Code)
Evaluation The initial evaluation consists of procedures to determine if the child is a child with a disability and to determine the educational needs of the child.	**OT 4.03** An occupational therapist alone or in collaboration with the occupational therapy assistant shall prepare an occupational therapy evaluation for each individual referred for occupational therapy services. The occupational therapist interprets the information gathered in the evaluation process. (WI Admin Code) **OT Framework:** Evaluation equals Occupational Profile plus Analysis of Occupational Performance
Decision 1. Does the child have an impairment? 2. Does the child need special education?	**OT 4.03** The occupational therapist interprets assessment data to identify facilitators and barriers to occupational performance.
IEP Development The IEP Team writes the IEP together. This includes deciding what services the child needs.	**OT 4.03** The occupational therapist • develops a plan that includes – objective and measurable goals with timeframe, – occupational therapy intervention approach based on theory and evidence, and – mechanisms for service delivery; • considers discharge needs and plans; • selects outcome measures; • makes a recommendation or referral to others as needed.
Placement IEP team decides on placement	**OT Framework:** what contexts support or inhibit desired outcomes?
Implementation LEA implements the IEP and placement.	**OT 4.03** The occupational therapist • determines types of occupational therapy interventions to be used and carries them out. • monitors the client's response according to ongoing assessment and reassessment.
Review and Re-evaluation IEP team reviews the IEP and placement at least annually. IEP team re-evaluates at least every three years, unless parents and school agree not to.	**OT 4.03** The occupational therapist • reevaluates plan relative to achieving targeted outcomes. • modifies the plan as needed. • determines the need for continuation, discontinuation, or referral.

The therapist must know about possible contraindications to intervention, as well as medical conditions that affect the child's current functional status.

To contact the physician or other professional directly, the therapist or other designated school employee must ask the child's parents for signed consent to release information. Therapists may contact only the specific agencies or individuals designated on the consent form and only during the period of time specified on the form. Schools must treat as confidential the written records that health care providers send to the school, or which therapists prepare from verbal information given by health care providers. School district employees may have access to those records only if they need them to comply with a requirement in federal or state law, or if the child's parent gives informed consent. (Chapter 146, Wis. Stats.)

Occasionally when therapists seek permission for communication with a physician, the parent responds that the child does not have a doctor, or the physician responds that he or she has not seen the child recently enough to provide relevant information. The therapist should seek assistance from the director of special education to work with the parent to obtain medical information, explaining that the district must provide safe and legal therapy. The school may be required to provide transportation or other assistance to the parents. The school district cannot deny related services to a child due to the difficulty in obtaining medical information. Figure 17 on the next page is a sample medical information worksheet that may clarify the exchange of information between therapists and physicians.

An evaluation must include an assessment of how occupational performance components and occupational performance contexts influence the individual's functional abilities and deficits in occupational performance areas.

Components of Occupational Therapy Evaluation

An OT conducting an evaluation in Wisconsin must consider an individual's medical, vocational, social, educational, and family status, as well as personal and family goals. The evaluation must include an assessment of how occupational performance components and occupational performance contexts influence the individual's functional abilities and deficits in occupational performance areas. The OT must evaluate and document occupational performance areas and components in the initial occupational therapy evaluation, periodically throughout intervention, and upon discontinuation of services. These requirements are part of the standards of practice that regulate all OTs and OTAs licensed to practice in Wisconsin. (OT 4.03(3)(b),(5)(b),(6)(b) and (6)(c), Wis. Admin Code)

An additional review of Figure 14 offers a reminder of the terms and concepts that relate to the components of occupational therapy evaluation. Occupational performance areas correspond to areas of occupation, those life activities in which individuals of all ages engage, such as "activities needed for learning and participating in the environment." (AOTA 2008) Occupational performance components correspond to performance skills, the features of what one does which rely on client factors and are often organized into performance patterns. Using Figure 14, it is clear to understand that examples of performance skills and patterns in school might be attending to instruction, remaining in a designated area, gathering materials for a task, and staying on task. Occupational performance contexts are the conditions in which the individual engages in activities of occupation. Context changes constantly, not only over a lifespan but also within a school day, as in going to and from school, participating in a class, or getting ready for bed. Because context is inseparable from performance areas and performance components, they too change. For example, consider Bill, a young, single male with a lifelong disability, who is developing a career. He is currently in physically accessible environments and has public transportation and wheelchair repair services available to him. Bill interacts with his context and environment to engage in occupation. If Bill were to move to a rural area, marry, or become seriously ill, the context of his occupational performance would change, and his current goals could lose relevance.

Occupational Profile

In the *Framework*, evaluation is the first step in the process of service delivery. Evaluation refers to the process of gathering information as a basis for making decisions. It is divided into two subsets: the occupational profile, and the analysis of occupational performance. The occupational profile is information that describes the client's background and perspective in order to determine client-centered goals and individualize intervention. It includes the kind of descriptive information that is often found in the *present level of academic achievement and functional performance* section of a child's IEP. To complete the occupational profile, the OT and OTA ask these questions:

- Who is the client?

- Why is the client seeking services?

- What occupations and activities are successful or are causing problems?

- What contexts support or inhibit desired outcomes?

- What is the client's occupational history?

- What are the client's priorities and targeted outcomes? (AOTA 2008)

For young children, some questions may be answered by parents, caregivers and teachers. Knippenberg and Hanft (2002) add questions that may be more relevant to children in educational environments:

- What does the student need to learn?

- What behaviors does a teacher expect and allow in the classroom?

- Where is the student successful?

- Where academically and socially across the school setting is this student struggling?

- What strategies have been tried and what was the child's response?

Figure 17 Sample Medical Information Worksheet

Consent to Obtain/Release of Information: _____
                                                                              date

To/From :_____
                                           agency or physician

(Attach copy of consent form)

Return to: _____
                                         district contact person

Child's name: _____ Date of Birth: _____

Parents: _____ Phone: _____

E-mail_____

Street Address:_____
                       street   city   ZIP code

Diagnosis/Etiology: _____

Date last seen by physician:_____

Physician's name: _____

Physician's address: _____
                        street   city   ZIP code

Medical Precautions (specify and/or list current medications if applicable)

— Seizure disorder _____

— Orthopedic concerns _____

— Surgeries (include past history)

    _____

    _____

    _____

    _____

— Shunted(include dates) _____

— Asthma or respiratory problems _____

— Allergies _____

— Visual impairment/Hearing impairment _____

— Neuromuscular condition (asymmetry, abnormal tone) _____

— Frequent ear infections _____

— Oral motor concerns that may affect feeding (include swallow deficits, food

    allergies, special diet, etc.) _____

    _____

— Other_____

Future Plans for:

— Surgical intervention _____

— Splinting/orthotics _____

— Equipment _____

— Medication changes _____

Additional precautions or medical information that might be pertinent to this child's school programming. _____

_____

_____

Therapist's Contact Documentation

Date	Therapist	**Contact Person** *How Contacted—Phone, Written, In Person*

Office of Student Services, School District of Waukesha. Adapted with permission.

As an IEP team member, the OT's review of existing information, described in chapter 3, may inform the occupational profile. In a school occupational therapy evaluation, OTs and OTAs gather information about a student's engagement in learning and assuming the student role, as well as other occupations of children and youth in educational environments. These occupations may include play, sports, activities of daily living, social participation, and preparation for adult occupations like careers, postsecondary schooling, relationships, and home management. (Moyers and Dale 2007)

Analysis of Occupational Performance

The occupational profile helps the OT to identify focal areas of occupation that she will address in the second part of evaluation, analysis of occupational performance. The therapist analyzes student performance by assessing contexts, activity demands, and client factors that influence performance skills and patterns in educational environments. Assessment refers to a specific tool, instrument, test or interaction that is used in the evaluation process. (Moyers and Dale 2007) It is defined in Chapter OT 1.02(1) Wis. Admin Code as "...a component part of the evaluation process, and means the process of determining the need for, nature of, and estimated time of treatment at different intervals during the treatment, determining needed coordination with or referrals to other disciplines, and documenting these activities." The following section describes a variety of assessment methods that OTs use to gather data for analysis of occupational performance in educational environments. The school OT interprets the information gathered in the evaluation process, (OT 4.03(3)(a), Wis. Admin Code) then formulates an occupational performance problem statement that describes the strengths and weaknesses of the child with respect to the patterns and routines of the school day and contextual supports and barriers to performance. Asher, I.E. (2007) in the references at the end of this chapter provides a comprehensive index of occupational therapy assessments in these categories:

> Performance in Areas of Occupation
> Performance Skills and Client Factors
> Performance Patterns and Contexts

Assessment Methods

The methods that an OT uses to analyze a child's occupational performance may include observation, interviews, records review, and the use of structured or standardized evaluative tools or techniques. (OT 4.03(3)(c), Wis. Admin Code) In best practice, an OT approaches evaluation in a collaborative manner. Collaborative evaluation means that the child's parent and the professional members of the educational team together set priorities about the environments and activities where they will assess the child's performance, and determine which team members will participate in each part of the assessment. (Rainforth and York-Barr 1997, 132)

It also means that the OT might not directly assess every occupational performance area and component in every relevant environment, but may gather

---

OTs and OTAs gather information about a student's engagement in learning and assuming the student role, as well as other occupations of children and youth in educational environments.

An OT uses observation, interviews, records review, and the use of structured or standardized evaluative tools or techniques.

information from parents, teachers, the child's records, and other service providers or persons in the child's life if the parent gave consent. With this approach, there may be more preparatory work because the members of the IEP team must plan ahead and coordinate their efforts, but they avoid duplication of data collection and are more likely to communicate throughout the evaluation. When the team prioritizes the order of activities and environments and identifies those that require an OT's perspective, the OT uses the most appropriate means of assessment. The therapist may perform the assessment alone, or collaborate with other team members. For instance, one team member could design a method of collecting data, while another carries it out. Tools may include any combination of informal and formal approaches, such as the following.

1. *Analysis of activity demands, observation, and recording of a baseline frequency of specific age-appropriate school activities in their naturally occurring contexts.* (Baumgart et al. 1982; Asher, 2007) This method is especially appropriate for analyzing a recurring aspect of a child's occupational performance that teachers and parents have identified as absent, emerging, or problematic. OT's often measure activities of daily living and social participation in this way and then rate them on a criterion-referenced instrument such as the *School Function Assessment* or a functional behavior assessment. This method provides a clear baseline measurement for the child's present level of academic achievement and functional performance in the IEP. It lends itself to accurate measurement of progress toward functional goals. The first step is a task analysis of the "aspects of an activity, which include the objects, space, social demands, sequencing or timing, required action, and required underlying client factors and body structures needed to carry out the activity." (AOTA 2008) From this, the OT can identify which activity demands are not being met, and record a baseline frequency of the aspects needing change. In *Functional Behavior Assessment: A Study Guide* (CESA 12 1999), the authors identify the following types and means of recording behavior.

   - Frequency or event recording. Generally the easiest and most accurate method of data collection, this is a count of how many times a specific behavior occurs during a given time period. It works best with behaviors that are discrete (have a clear start and stop, take about the same amount of time whenever they occur, can be distinguished from another event), rather than continuous (not as easy to tell when it stops or starts).

   - Interval recording. The observer divides the time (generally less than one hour) into equal intervals (probably no more than 30 seconds each), and then records whether or not the behavior occurs during each interval. Simple symbols (+ and -) and a timing device, usually a watch with a second hand, are used.

The first step is a task analysis. From this, the OT can identify which activity demands are not being met, and record a baseline frequency of the aspects needing change.

- Time-sampling. Similar to interval recording, in this method the observer looks only momentarily in random or unequal intervals. The advantage of this method is that the observer can do other things along with the data collection. The disadvantage is that it is possible to miss a behavior with longer intervals and obtain less accurate data.

- Duration recording. This is a measure of how long a particular behavior lasts. It works best with skills or behaviors that must be maintained over time, such as staying seated or eating a meal. It is also useful for measuring decreases in behaviors that interfere with function.

- Latency recording. This is a way to document the amount of time between behaviors. The interval between the teacher giving a direction and the student complying with the request is an example of latency recording. Another example is how long a student must rest before resuming an activity.

- Scatter plot. Over a week, the observer records occurrences of the behavior on a time grid (such as the days of the week divided into 15- or 30-minute time intervals). Scatter plots can determine when and where to collect data about behavior, and, when charted, that information can reveal behavioral patterns.

- Antecedent–Behavior–Consequence. This is typically a narrative account of the environmental events that precede observable behavior (antecedents), an objective description of the behavior, and an account of events that follow that behavior (consequences).

Analysis of the activities, people, and communication that make up a naturally occurring environment or routine allows therapists to look at how the environment or the actions of others may initiate or reinforce performance.

2. *Analysis of the activities, people, and communication that make up a naturally occurring environment or routine.* (Griswold 1994, McWilliam and Clingenpeel 2003) Occupational performance is also influenced by context and environment, as well as the more commonly assessed client factors and activity demands. The recording method of antecedent-behavior-consequence described above allows therapists to begin to look at how the environment or the actions of others may initiate or reinforce performance. OTs use this type of approach when they observe the effects of the sensory environment of the classroom upon a child's behavior. A therapist could also interview a parent, teacher or student about the routines of a typical day at home or school to find out which routines are successful and which are not.

3. *Experimentation with tasks or environments by controlling or manipulating some element to determine a cause-effect relationship.* (Asher 2007, Silverman et al. 2000) Assessment may include changing an aspect of an activity or trying equipment to see if occupational performance improves. Assistive technology assessment is a familiar example of this approach. In

an initial evaluation, the OT may measure a child's ability to meet classroom expectations for producing written assignments without the use of an assistive device to derive a baseline. Assessment may proceed to trying devices that promise to improve performance over time, such as an electronic keyboard or voice-activated computer input software. The therapist will measure the results of each trial in order to select the most appropriate device for intervention.

4. *Measurement using an appropriate instrument selected or developed for the purpose.* This method is probably the most familiar but typically measures only client factors of occupational performance. This category includes paper-and-pencil objective tests, performance tests, work samples, projective techniques, inventories, rating scales, mechanical devices, or computer programs. (Asher 2007) The use of standardized instruments is discussed in more detail below. Any evaluation materials, procedures, or tests that are used must

- be administered in the child's native language or other mode of communication and in the form most likely to yield accurate information on what the child knows and can do academically, developmentally and functionally.

- not be racially or culturally discriminatory.

- be used for the purposes for which they are valid and reliable.

- have normative data for the child's characteristics, such as age and disability, or else be expressed in descriptive rather than quantitative terms.

- reflect the child's aptitude or achievement level and not the child's impaired sensory, manual, or speaking skills, unless those are the factors the test is designed to measure.

- be administered by trained and knowledgeable personnel in accordance with the instructions provided by their producer. (OT 4.03, Wis. Admin Code, and 115.782, Wis. Stats.)

Use of Standardized Instruments

Standardized instruments are those in which the procedure, apparatus and scoring are fixed so that the same procedures are followed exactly, each time that the test is administered. (Cronbach 1990) Standardized interviews, standardized observations and standardized tests all may fall into this category. Standardized assessments can be norm-referenced or criterion-referenced. Norm-referenced assessments compare results to the scores that are expected from a comparable group of typical subjects. Criterion-referenced assessments compare results to criteria. (Asher 2007) An OT cannot conduct a comprehensive evaluation of a child's performance in areas of occupation using only standardized, norm-

An OT cannot conduct a comprehensive evaluation of a child's performance in areas of occupation using only standardized, norm-referenced tests.

referenced tests. Such tests, however, can provide objective and measurable information, when used correctly. The therapist should report normative scores for such tests only in the following circumstances: if the child's age is within the available norms, if the test is valid for the child's disability and culture, if the therapist administers the test in the child's native language, and if the therapist follows the standardized procedure for administering the test. These criteria will yield valid normative scores that are useful only if the therapist can relate them to the child's functional performance in the naturally occurring school environment. A child's score on any given test or tests neither qualifies nor disqualifies that child for school occupational therapy. It is the overall IEP team evaluation and program planning that leads to an IEP team decision of whether occupational therapy is required to assist the child to benefit from special education.

Reporting Results

The OT communicates evaluation results to the referral source and to the appropriate persons in the facility and community. (OT 4.03(3)(f), Wis. Admin Code) At the IEP team meeting that concludes the evaluation process, the therapist contributes to the pool of information that everyone brings to the meeting. The team uses the collective information to determine if the child meets the criteria for one or more of the impairments identified in state law. If the team identifies an impairment, members determine if the child needs special education.

OTs are required to prepare an evaluation for each individual referred for occupational therapy services and to document the results.

The IEP team develops a collaborative evaluation report that documents the determination of the child's area of impairment, if any, and the information that was used to make that determination. If the child meets the criteria for one or more impairments, the IEP team also documents whether or not the child needs special education. Since 2006, IDEA and state law have not required individual IEP team members to write a summary of evaluation findings but to accept the collectively produced document. OTs, however, are required by Chapter OT 4.03(3), Wis. Admin Code to prepare an evaluation for each individual referred for occupational therapy services and to document the results in the individual's record. The report must indicate the specific evaluation tools and methods that the therapist used, as well as the status of the individual's occupational performance areas and performance components. The report is most useful if it is written in terms that are understandable to parents and other IEP team members and relates to the child's ability to function in academic and non-academic areas in school. The report should help the IEP team answer these questions:

- What is the child's functional performance at school?

- How does the child's disability affect his or her involvement and progress in the general education curriculum or age-appropriate activities?

- What are the child's strengths?

- What does the child need to learn?

- What are the parent's concerns?

The Guide to Occupational Therapy Practice (Moyers and Dale, 2007) illustrates a documentation structure that lends itself to addressing the evaluation components of the *Framework*, the occupational therapy licensure law requirements in Wisconsin, and the information needs of the IEP team. The structure includes

- identifying information about the child and relevant information from the occupational profile.

- evaluation tools and assessment methods used.

- analysis of occupational performance, beginning with identification of strengths and weaknesses of performance in areas of occupation and including baseline frequency of performance in specific age-appropriate school activities that emerge as areas of concern in their naturally occurring contexts.

- identification of occupational performance skills, performance patterns, client factors, activity demands, environments and/or contexts that interfere with or support occupational performance in areas of concern.

- identification of factors that are amenable to intervention.

- recommendations for the IEP team to consider such as occupational therapy intervention, support to teachers, or supplementary aids and services.

If the OT is excused from attending the IEP team meeting, his or her evaluation report may include a recommendation of the nature, frequency, and amount of occupational therapy.

The inclusion of baseline frequencies of performance will assist the IEP team in writing annual goals that they can measure in the same terms as the statement of present levels. If test scores are obtained, they can be included in the selected performance skills and client factors. If the OT is excused from attending the IEP team meeting, as described in chapter 3, his or her evaluation report may also include a recommendation concerning the nature, frequency, and amount of the occupational therapy that the therapist believes the child needs.

Other School Occupational Therapy Evaluations

In addition to participating in a child's initial evaluation to determine eligibility for special education and educational needs, OTs often participate in a child's periodic reevaluation of special education and related service needs, as well as in specialized evaluations such as functional behavioral assessments.

Re-evaluation

The IEP team conducts a reevaluation of each child with a disability at least once every three years and no more than once a year, unless the school district and the parent agree otherwise. Other reasons for additional reevaluations include a request by the child's parent or teacher, or when changes occur in the educational or related services needs of the child, including improved academic achievement and functional performance. (34 CFR 300.303(a)(1)

When the IEP team that includes an OT conducts a three-year reevaluation of a child, the occupational therapy reevaluation will include

- an assessment of the child's present levels of functional performance in occupational performance areas, components, and contexts. (Chapter OT 4.03(5)(b), Wis. Admin Code)

- a comparison of the child's status at the previous evaluation to the child's present levels of functional performance.

- a review of strategies and adaptations that the child has tried, those found to be successful, and supporting data.

- any recommendations for continuation or initiation of specific strategies and adaptations.

The OT assesses a child's progress periodically or continuously during intervention, using any of the methods discussed above. The therapist may be responsible for collecting data and documenting progress toward IEP goals according to the procedures and schedule on the IEP, or may provide information to another team member who will report the progress to the child's parent. When a school district seeks third-party payment for occupational therapy, the therapist follows the requirements for assessing and reporting progress as required by the payer, in addition to those required by special education law. Prior to the annual IEP meeting, the OT summarizes the data collected during the year on progress toward IEP goals and any changes that have occurred in the treatment plan. The OT may conduct additional assessments for the purpose of establishing baselines and developing IEP goals at the meeting without obtaining parental consent.

Functional Behavioral Assessment

Functional behavioral assessment (FBA) is a process conducted by an IEP team for the purpose of identifying (1) the function of a child's behavior; (2) the variables that influence the behavior; and (3) the components of an effective behavioral intervention plan (BIP). (CESA 12 1999) If a child's behavior impedes the child's learning or that of others, the IEP team must consider the use of positive behavioral interventions and supports (PBIS) to address the behavior. (34 CFR 300.324 (a) (2)) FBA is based on applied behavioral analysis and is a foundation for determining positive behavioral interventions. It is a process that the IEP team uses to

- identify and define a specific, observable behavior.

- determine the antecedent, that is, what precedes the behavior of concern.

- identify the consequence, or that which follows the target behavior.

The team should document a specific behavior in a way that anyone reading the statement could identify the behavior when it occurs. Terms that are subject to interpretation can lead to inconsistent implementation of a behavioral plan. Antecedents may include external factors such as settings, tasks, people, activities, or events, or internal factors such as neurological or medical

OTs provide critical observations and contributions to the functional behavioral assessment process and the development of positive behavioral intervention plans.

conditions. Consequences may include what the student does, what other students do, what teachers do or other adults do after the behavior occurs.

OTs provide critical observations and contributions to the FBA process and the development of positive behavioral intervention plans. In addition to bringing an understanding of neurology and medical conditions to the team, OTs attend to performance patterns, activity demands, contextual factors and environmental features of which other school staff may not be aware. For example, the motor demands of an activity or the sensory impact of a room or a teacher's voice may be antecedents to a behavior that interferes with learning. Prevention of the behavior through manipulation of antecedents, intervention through the use of self-regulatory strategies, and skill building by increasing self-awareness may be ways that OTs can contribute to PBIS for students and capacity building for teachers.

Intervention

Intervention refers to the skilled actions that the OT and OTA take to help the child meet his IEP goals. (AOTA 2008, 652) It is the step in the occupational therapy process that takes place after the IEP team writes occupational therapy into a child's IEP and sets a date for implementing services. The first phase of intervention is planning. The OT meets the program planning requirements described in Chapter OT 4.03(4), Wis. Admin Code, by participating in the IEP team meetings to develop each child's IEP, as well as by writing a separate occupational therapy treatment plan for each child as required by Chapter PI 11.24, Wis. Admin Code. The OT may collaborate with the OTA, the teacher, the student or others to derive a treatment plan from the functional, age-appropriate outcomes in the child's IEP. The therapist uses the treatment plan as a tool to guide specific interventions so they remain synchronized with the IEP, and thus with the provision of special education and other related services. The plan also helps to guide others who may be implementing the child's occupational therapy, such as an OTA or an OT in another school if the child transfers. The treatment plan may take various forms, depending on the model of service delivery that the team considers most appropriate and the strategies that the OT and teacher select. Occupational therapy treatment plans commonly include short-term goals that are written to define the expected change in occupational performance as a result of the planned intervention. Change may take the form of

The OT meets program planning requirements by participating in the IEP team meetings to develop each child's IEP, as well as by writing a separate occupational therapy treatment plan for each child.

- increased frequency, duration, consistency, quality or safety of performance.

- decreased levels of assistance, time, errors, or behaviors that interfere with performance.

- new performance. (Moyers & Dale 2007)

The planned intervention approaches and methods are recorded on the treatment plan. The OT alone may change the treatment plan as the child's needs change, as the intervention is not part of the child's IEP. Components of the treatment plan that are directly from the IEP, such as IEP goals and amount and frequency of service may not be changed without an IEP team meeting or the agreement of the parent and school to change the IEP without a meeting. Appendix B provides examples of school occupational therapy treatment plans. Occupational therapy treatment plans are generally considered patient health care records under Chapter 146, Wis. Stats. They may be stored in the therapist's secure files and should be shared with parents at their request.

Principles of Intervention

School OTs base their intervention with a child with a disability on several principles from IDEA and occupational therapy practice. These include the following:

- the child has access to the general curriculum in order to meet the educational standards that apply to all children in the school district. (34 CFR s. 300.39(b)(3)(ii))

- the child is educated with children who are nondisabled to the maximum extent appropriate. (34 CFR s. 300.114(a)(2)(i))

- special education and related services are designed to meet the unique needs of the child and prepare him or her for further education, employment, and independent living. (34 CFR s.300.1(a))

- related services to be provided to the child or on behalf of the child are based on peer-reviewed research to the extent practicable. (34 CFR s. 300.320(a)(4))

- occupation includes activities of daily living, instrumental activities of daily living, education, social participation, play, leisure and work. (Moyers and Dale 2007)

- the OT focuses on changing factors in the client, activity, context and environments, performance skills, or performance patterns in order for the child to achieve health and participation in life through engagement in occupations. (AOTA 2008, 656)

Children with Speech and Language Impairments

Occasionally an IEP team questions whether or not a child who meets the criteria for speech and language impairment and needs special education to improve articulation may also receive occupational therapy that is unrelated to articulation or oral motor skills. IDEA explicitly states that special education and related services are based on the identified needs of the child and not on the disability category in which the child is classified. (34 CFR Part 300.8, Analysis and Comments) Types of services, such as occupational therapy, are not restricted to children in specific categories.

Once the IEP team determines that a child meets eligibility in any one of the impairment categories and needs special education, the team will develop goals related to the child's academic and functional needs. They should consider all of

IDEA explicitly states that special education and related services are based on the identified needs of the child and not on the disability category in which the child is classified.

the child's needs that affect educational progress and participation, but may prioritize the needs that will be addressed in the IEP. For a child with a speech and language impairment, the team may decide to write goals for areas of need in addition to speech, such as written communication, social skills, mobility, or behavior. The IEP will describe the special education services needed to implement the goals, including the amount, location and duration. A special education teacher other than the speech therapist may provide these special education services. If the team decides that occupational therapy is required to assist the child to benefit from special education, they will list it as a related service. It is important for the team to discuss other reasonable alternatives to special education and occupational therapy, such as regular education program modifications or supplementary aids and services. If the IEP team members follow the process described in chapter 3, postponing a decision about the need for occupational therapy until goals are written and special education services are determined, they then can ask if occupational therapy is required to assist the child to benefit from special education in meeting the goals or ensuring participation. An occupational therapy evaluation that identified skill deficits does not automatically mean that the child requires occupational therapy; rather, it is up to each child's IEP team to determine the special education and related services that will address the child's unique needs in order for the child to receive a free, appropriate public education.

Intervention Approaches

The *Framework* identifies five categories of intervention (AOTA 2008):

The Framework identifies five categories of intervention.

1. *Create, promote.* Depending on the district's job description, this approach may be an incidental or optional category of occupational therapy intervention in schools, as it is not specific to individuals with disabilities. An OT may provide services that are likely to improve occupational performance for all students in a school. In educational terminology, this approach is often called a *universal intervention.* Examples are consulting on an ergonomic seating plan, contributing to the design of a playground, developing a backpack awareness program, mentoring teachers in a cognitive-sensory program for self-regulation, and assisting in the development of a school wide handwriting curriculum. Hanft & Shepherd (2008) call this approach *system support* and describes is as "an opportunity to apply one's professional wisdom and experience to develop programs and policies to build the capacity of a school district and its education teams."

2. *Establish, restore.* With this approach, the OT's intent is to establish or restore a child's performance skills or patterns, or change client factors such as muscle strength. The OT uses this type of intervention to prepare the child for more active performance in occupations. Examples are exercise and therapeutic practice of a motor skill. Restorative approaches are incomplete and frequently ineffective without facilitating a transfer of the targeted skill to the performance of occupations and activities in natural environments.

3. *Maintain.* The purpose of this approach is to ensure that a child's occupational performance remains at a functional level. It is often used when the child is at risk for losing function or when therapeutic goals have been achieved and an intense level of intervention is no longer required.

4. *Modify and Compensate.* In this approach, the OT develops strategies for task or activity performance by

- teaching alternative strategies for accomplishing the desired outcome.

- altering the activity or the activity demands.

- adapting the context or environment in which the child performs.

- improving the child's performance through assistive devices.

5. *Prevent.* Using this approach, the OT takes action to prevent barriers to occupational performance, such as physical deterioration or emotional distress. These preventive actions frequently include positioning, task adaptation, or modification of the environment. They are often directed toward ensuring physical safety or positive behavior.

Evidence-Based Practices in Intervention

Occupational therapy literature commonly describes evidence-based practice as a process of reviewing published research to gather the most reliable evidence about the effectiveness of selected interventions or practice patterns, that is, the way in which intervention is implemented, and applying that evidence to choices made in practice. (Holm 2000; Dysart and Tomlin 2002) An evidence-based occupational therapy practice uses research evidence together with clinical knowledge and reasoning to make decisions about interventions that are effective for a specific client. (Law and Baum 1998) In defining scientifically based research, IDEA refers to section 9101(37) of the ESEA, also known as No Child Left Behind:

Scientifically based research—(a) Means research that involves the application of rigorous, systematic, and objective procedures to obtain reliable and valid knowledge relevant to education activities and programs; and (b) Includes research that—

(1) Employs systematic, empirical methods that draw on observation or experiment;

(2) Involves rigorous data analyses that are adequate to test the stated hypotheses and justify the general conclusions drawn;

(3) Relies on measurements or observational methods that provide reliable and valid data across evaluators and observers, across multiple measurements and observations, and across studies by the same or different investigators;

(4) Is evaluated using experimental or quasi-experimental designs in which individuals, entities, programs, or activities are assigned to different conditions and with appropriate controls to evaluate the effects of the condition of interest, with a preference for random-assignment experiments,

An evidence-based occupational therapy practice uses research evidence together with clinical knowledge and reasoning to make decisions about interventions that are effective for a specific client.

or other designs to the extent that those designs contain within-condition or across-condition controls;

(5) Ensures that experimental studies are presented in sufficient detail and clarity to allow for replication or, at a minimum, offer the opportunity to build systematically on their findings; and

(6) Has been accepted by a peer-reviewed journal or approved by a panel of independent experts through a comparably rigorous, objective, and scientific review.

By this definition, the availability of scientifically based research on interventions used by OTs with children is very limited. Evidence-based practice urges service providers to ask whether an intervention really does work in controlled trials rather than accepting that it *should* work on the basis of an understanding of its neurological or physiological principles. Evidence-based practice also places less value on expert opinion that is not supported by scientific research. A hierarchy of evidence that is commonly cited in the literature includes these levels from the work of D.L. Sackett et al. 2000:

I   Strong evidence from at least one systematic review of multiple, well-designed, randomized controlled trials

II   Strong evidence from at least one properly designed randomized controlled trial of appropriate size

III Evidence from well-designed trials without randomization, single group pre-post, cohort, time series, or match case-controlled studies

IV   Evidence from well-designed non-experimental studies from more than one center or research group

V   Opinions of respected authorities, based on clinical evidence, descriptive studies, or reports of expert committees

To begin building an evidence-based occupational therapy practice, Cope (2005) recommends that the therapist

- pose a researchable question.

- search the literature for the best evidence available.

- critically appraise the study's validity.

- integrate the evidence into the decision about intervention.

The evidence reviewed should help the therapist decide whether to start an intervention not currently in use, or whether to reconsider, modify or continue an intervention currently in use.

The evidence reviewed should help the therapist decide whether to start an intervention not currently in use, or whether to reconsider, modify or continue an intervention currently in use. Questions the therapist should ask about the evidence include

- How much evidence exists?

- How much evidence is needed to make this decision?

- Is the available evidence credible by IDEA standards?

- Can the original program design of a studied intervention be implemented with fidelity in the educational context?

- Does the evidence support or refute providing the intervention for the child in question with the desired outcomes?

In many instances, the term *evidence-based practice* reflects the efficacy of theory-based interventions in which the therapist directly engages the child in order to establish or restore a child's performance skills or patterns, or change client factors. Evidence-based practice also applies to the way in which intervention is implemented. In order for intervention to be relevant to children's needs in school, gains resulting from occupational therapy must become part of the child's daily routines. (Dunn and Westman 1995) Making intervention part of the child's routine requires that the OT support others who have daily contact with the child; collaborate to create therapeutic environments where children are working, learning, or playing; and adapt tasks and materials to enable the child to perform successfully. The evidence that supports integrating interventions into daily routines arises primarily from two key practices, inclusive education and collaboration.

The first key practice, inclusive education, refers to "placement and membership of students with disabilities in general education." (Rainforth and York-Barr 1997, 9) This principle, legally known as least restrictive environment or LRE, has been an important element of IDEA since its inception. LRE means that "to the maximum extent appropriate, children with disabilities, including children in public or private institutions or other care facilities, are educated with children who are nondisabled; and special classes, separate schooling, or other removal of children with disabilities from the regular educational environment occurs only if the nature or severity of the disability is such that education in regular classes with the use of supplementary aids and services cannot be achieved satisfactorily." (CFR § 300.114) Education policy and court cases, as well as an increasing body of research, support inclusion in the general curriculum and the regular education classroom with appropriate supports as the IEP team's first consideration for a child with a disability. Students with disabilities who have been educated with peers without disabilities in inclusive settings have shown higher levels of social interaction, social competence, communication, skill acquisition, grade and test achievement, and school attendance. (McGregor and Vogelsberg 1998, Rea et al. 2002) McWilliam and Scott (2003) report that children generalize more following in-class than pull-out therapy. Occupational therapy models that emphasize engagement, participation and mastery in daily activities that occur in natural contexts assist the OT to provide services in the LRE for the child. An integrated therapy model is not an opportunity to reduce staff time or numbers. Effective use of integrated occupational therapy requires as much, and possibly more time initially, as a traditional direct service model. (Dunn 1991)

In order for intervention to be relevant to children's needs in school, gains resulting from occupational therapy must become part of the child's daily routines.

A second key practice, school-based collaboration, is defined by Hanft and Shepherd (2008) as "an interactive team process that focuses education, related service, family and student partners on the academic and nonacademic performance and participation of all students in school." Studies in the literature of occupational therapy report increased effectiveness of collaborative models among general educators, special educators and related service providers compared to isolated service provision. (Dunn 1990; Giangreco 1986) McWilliam and Scott (2003) report that over time, both families and therapists preferred integrated, in-class models of service provision. They found that when therapy is provided in the classroom, teachers and specialists consult with each other four times as much as they do when a child is pulled out for therapy.

Measuring Individual Student Outcomes

Acknowledging the limited availability of Level I and II research that is relevant to school occupational therapy, Swinth et al. (2007) recommend that school OTs use systematic data-based decision-making to help inform their interventions. Sarracino (2002) discusses the difference as well as the link between applying evidence-based interventions in daily practice and measuring functional outcomes for individual students who receive special education and occupational therapy. The ongoing measurement of student outcomes in relation to intervention is often called *progress monitoring*. Progress monitoring is defined as a scientifically based practice that is used to assess students' academic performance and evaluate the effectiveness of instruction. (National Center on Student Progress Monitoring 2010)

The ongoing measurement of student outcomes in relation to intervention is often called progress monitoring.

In a collaborative school community, progress monitoring is used as part of a school-wide approach to education of all students. It is based on three key questions:

1. What do we expect all students to be able to know and do?

2. How do we know if students are meeting expectations?

3. What do we do if students are not meeting expectations?

The way a school community answers these questions is important to an OT providing individual service to a child with a disability and the child's teachers. Typically, a school district will have academic standards similar to the Wisconsin Model Academic Standards, (DPI 2010) and a curriculum that is aligned to the standards. A district that uses progress monitoring will develop benchmarks that identify proficiency that students need to achieve at certain points over time, and indicators of the critical skills that need to be measured. The collection of performance data on all students reveals if instruction and universal options benefit all students. (Dohrn, et al., 2006) Progress monitoring is not limited to academic skills, but is critical to fostering acquisition of social, emotional and behavioral skills. Standards, benchmarks, indicators and high quality instruc-tional options in these areas provide educators with a systematic way to improve student learning. Since students with disabilities are included in the general education curriculum and environment, they benefit from the instruction and intervention options that are available to all students. The service that an OT provides to a child with a disability should complement, supplement, inform and be informed by the instruction and intervention that the general education teacher and special education teacher provide to the child.

An example of an application of these principles to student handwriting skills may help to clarify their relevance to school occupational therapy. In a 2000 study of Wisconsin school OTs and PTs, the primary reason OTs reported making recommendations for therapy was written work; 92 percent of OTs surveyed selected this area. (Chiang and Rylance 2000) One group of OTs in a Wisconsin school district received increasing numbers of referrals for students whose handwriting did not meet teacher expectations. Many of the children referred did not have identified disabilities. The therapists surveyed fifteen first- and second-grade teachers in the district and found that 70 percent of the teachers were dissatisfied with their knowledge base for teaching handwriting. (Flood, et al. 2001) They did not know how to work on letter formation or correct poor writing patterns, yet expected students to complete writing tasks in a specified amount of time (as in question 1 above, what do we expect all students to be able to know and do?) Following a review of literature as well as instruction and mentoring by several experts in handwriting instruction, the therapists randomly selected three of the fifteen classrooms as a control group. They gave a pretest on letter formation to all 278 first- and second-grade students in all fifteen classrooms (as in question 2, how do we know if students are meeting expectations?) The therapists then applied a universal intervention to the study group of twelve classrooms. They provided each classroom with 30 sessions of direct handwriting instruction, designed to educate the students and model instruction for the teacher. They also gave handwriting activity kits to each classroom and teacher incentives to attend two in-services on handwriting instruction (as in question 3, what do we do if students are not meeting expectations?). Post-testing showed that students in the study group made consistent improvement in all areas assessed, compared to some improvement and some worsening of performance in the control group. Of equal interest was the change in teacher knowledge and receptiveness. Teacher dissatisfaction with their knowledge of teaching handwriting dropped from 70 percent to 33 percent (teachers in the control group were included). They gained confidence and interest in incorporating handwriting instruction into writing assignments. Both the teachers and the therapists gained knowledge about which problems can be improved by differential instruction, and which required interventions to change or compensate for client factors. Teachers became aware of discrepancies in terminology, materials, and strategies across grade levels and classrooms and implemented greater consistency. Asher (2006) found a similar effect in a review of the practices of 47 elementary school teachers in teaching handwriting.

One approach to progress monitoring, general outcome measurement (GOM) identifies a single general task that provides an indication of change in the general outcome desired and then repeatedly measures performance on that task

The service that an OT provides should complement, supplement, inform and be informed by the instruction and intervention that the general education teacher and special education teacher provide to the child.

over time to gauge the extent of change. (Deno 2009) Research evidence supporting the reliability and validity of the GOM approach is extensive, and GOM is widely used in schools for progress monitoring. The approach involves frequent, brief, repeated sampling of student performance on a single core task from the curriculum.

A second approach to progress monitoring, mastery monitoring, uses task analysis of a desired academic outcome like reading proficiency into small component skills and then measures progress in attaining mastery of each of those small component skills. Mastery monitoring measures how many and which steps in a process a student masters compared with established criteria. Carlson (2008) described the steps of mastery monitoring used by OTs and physical therapists (PTs) in Iowa:

1. defining the behavior

2. selecting a measurement strategy

3. documenting the current level of function

4. setting goals and practice

5. charting

6. developing a decision-making plan

Goal Attainment Scaling is a way to measure progress that is meaningful and functional but often challenging to assess using standardized instruments.

A practical method for evaluating student progress toward a goal is Goal Attainment Scaling (GAS). Originally developed in the field of mental health (Kiresuk and Sherman 1968), GAS has been used with success to evaluate effectiveness of programs in psychotherapy, mental health, education, rehabilitation, and occupational therapy. (Ottenbacher and Cusick 1990; Mailloux et al. 2007) It is a way to measure progress that is meaningful and functional but often challenging to assess using standardized instruments. For example, parents and teachers may seek occupational therapy for their children for reasons such as social participation and self-regulation of behavior. In a study by Cohn (2001), parents reported that they valued improvements in their children's sense of self-worth following occupational therapy intervention more than they valued improved abilities, recognizing that improved abilities and engagement in activities contributed to feelings of self-worth. GAS measures individual changes in complex occupational performance over a short time with a high degree of sensitivity. (Mailloux, et al., 2007)

The process consists of the procedures described below for a child who has an IEP.

1. The IEP team defines the child's current status in the target skill or behavior and determines a target goal.

2. The team or relevant staff develops a continuum of operationally defined behavioral benchmarks that provide steps toward the goal.

3. The staff scales the benchmarks using a seven-point scale ranging from -3 to +3. The range of benchmarks corresponds to the best possible outcome (+3), no change (0) or worst possible outcome (-3). The benchmarks must be clearly defined so that observers will agree on when the behavior occurs. (Dohrn, et al. 2006) The original five-point scale used by Kiresuk and Sherman (1968) ranged from -2 to +2. Whichever scale is used, it should be used consistently with all students so that comparison of interventions over time is possible. It is important to set the child's present level of function at 0 so that possible regression can be captured.

4. The staff monitors the child's performance daily or weekly by graphing the number value that best describes the performance at that data point. (Dohrn, et al. 2006)

5. The staff evaluates the student outcomes and process, and develops next steps.

It is important to assess whether or not the intervention was implemented with fidelity. Fidelity refers to providing the intervention in a way that compares favorably with the original design of the evidence-based practice. Reliability can be increased by including multiple measurement periods, training the staff in specific progress monitoring practices, and developing explicit definitions or examples of the child's performance. (Ottenbacher and Cusick 1990) Guiding questions for this phase of evaluation are:

- Did we teach or intervene with what we agreed upon, assess what we agreed to assess, and follow the intervention and assessment guidelines?

- Did we provide the intervention with the planned frequency or exposure?

- Is the intervention evidence-based?

- Are we being true to the intention of the intervention as designed?

- Does the assessment measure what we say we are measuring?

The staff should look at the trend in the data and decide if it warrants continuation of the intervention. Figure 18 on the next page is a example worksheet that uses the GAS process and can serve as a model. Therapists can use raw benchmark scores to evaluate individual goals. Ottenbacher and Cusick (1990) provide an explanation of how to evaluate a student's overall progress in multiple goals, using a mathematical formula and prioritizing goals.

Common Areas of School Occupational Therapy Intervention

School personnel commonly request occupational therapy services when a child has difficulty with written communication skills, and a growing body of evidence is available to guide effective collaborative practices in this area. Wisconsin school OTs who were surveyed on the nature of their work reported recommending intervention for children in these major activities. (Chiang and Rylance 2000)

- Written work: 92 percent of OTs surveyed

- Computer and equipment use: 63.2 percent

- Material Use: 61.8 percent

- Manipulation with movement: 52.0 percent

- Eating and drinking: 44.0 percent%

- Maintaining and changing position: 43.2 percent

- Behavior regulation: 40.8 percent

- Adaptations: 31.6 percent

- Task behavior and completion: 28.0 percent

- Functional communication, socialization, hygiene, personal care awareness and safety: 21 to 25 percent

Written work, computer and equipment use, material use, and manipulation with movement. These are high-frequency activities in the occupational performance area of education. They are often characterized as fine motor skills, but in fact they involve a number of performance skills and client factors, such as

- posture, neuromusculoskeletal and movement-related functions.

- process skills, including organization of space and time.

- attention, sequencing, perception and other mental functions.

- sensory functions such as vision, touch, and body position.

Baker (1999) identified variables of motor learning as the use of feedback and practice as well as visual learning, mental practice, motivation, duration and frequency of practice sessions, and part or whole transfer. Feedback is both intrinsic, as in the integration of sensations from muscles and joints, and extrinsic, as in seeing the outcome of the movement. When applying motor learning research to classroom activities, the occupational therapy practitioner views the child as a problem-solver who needs to experience motor challenges that require the same sort of processing, as well as outcome, as functional motor goals. To facilitate processing during practice, the OT and the classroom teacher design random presentation of various tasks and variability within a task, and teach the child how to estimate his or her own performance based on intrinsic and extrinsic feedback. They plan how to reduce feedback from adults systematically, to encourage the child's independence. By planning and implementing the child's program in collaboration with the teacher, the OT ensures that practice occurs throughout the child's school day. "Practice that is plentiful in quantity and variety appears to enhance motor learning, particularly if the child is allowed to practice various skills in a random versus blocked fashion. The natural variability of tasks and contexts in the classroom provides an opportunity for the child to practice with variability that may be used to strengthen motor schema." (Baker 1999)

Written work, computer and equipment use, material use, and manipulation with movement are often characterized as fine motor skills, but in fact they involve a number of performance skills and client factors.

Figure 18 Example Goal Attainment Scaling Worksheet

Baseline in target behavior: Able to play alone with toys for two to three minutes; when other children are present, cannot share or interact with toys without adult assistance but bangs toys on floor or throws them at other children.	**+3** **Best possible outcome**	Without adult assistance, shares with another child and interacts with toys without banging or throwing them five times per day for 10 minutes.
	+2 **Much improved over baseline behavior**	Without adult assistance, shares with another child without physical aggression, five times per day for 5 minutes.
	+1 **More than baseline behavior**	When another child is present and without adult assistance, interacts with toys without banging or throwing them five times per day for 3 minutes.
Target goal: Share with another child and interact with toys without banging or throwing them, without adult assistance five times per day for 10 minutes.	**0** **No change in behavior (baseline)**	Plays alone with toys for 2-3 minutes; with other children present, cannot share or interact with toys without adult assistance but bangs toys on floor or throws them at other children.
	-1 **Less than baseline behavior**	Plays alone with toys for less than 2 minutes.
Intervention period: 20 sessions	**-2** **Much less than baseline behavior**	Requires adult assistance to play with toys when no other children are present
	-3 **Worst possible outcome**	Does not interact with toys. Engages in hitting or kicking others or screaming when other children are playing nearby.

Activity demands, environments and context influence a child's performance in these educational occupations. For example, a child who may produce legible handwriting during an untimed practice session may not do so when time limits, distractions, or testing conditions are present. Some level IV and V evidence as described by D.L. Sackett is available that supports the effectiveness of occupational therapy intervention in improving performance in these school activities. (Swinth, et al. 2007)

Eating and drinking. Children with severe disabilities may have educational needs related to eating. Eating is usually part of the school day for all children, and a child with a disability may be unable to participate in this activity without special education and related services. If a child has IEP goals related to eating, it is likely that a number of people, including a school OT, are involved in the development of strategies to implement these goals. School staff, parents, and medical personnel must clarify their roles related to a child's eating needs in school.

PI 11.24(9)(c) Wis. Admin Code states, "The school occupational therapist must have medical information regarding a child before the child receives occupational therapy. " The basis of this part of state law is to ensure that school OTs have sufficient knowledge about risk factors and medical interventions in order to provide safe intervention to a child. Because problems related to swallowing as well as nutritional intake can be life-threatening for some children, it is critical for school districts to obtain medical authorization for feeding children who have not yet begun oral feeding or have

- frequent respiratory illnesses.

- weight loss or poor weight gain.

- crying or resistance when food approaches the mouth.

- a history of dehydration.

- frequent gagging, choking, or coughing either with food, liquid or their own secretions. (Clark 1992)

A report from a swallow study or clearance from a physician based on a swallow study is the most definitive information related to safe oral feeding. The IEP team, including the parent, may consider developing an individualized health plan with assistance from the school nurse, along with the IEP if the child's feeding needs warrant detail that all involved personnel need to know.

Each child's program must be based on individual needs. In general, if the activity is still in the therapeutic phase when the judgment of an OT or OTA is required, the therapist will feed the child. (AOTA 2009) If oral feeding is a safe, learned skill that only requires routine physical assistance such as bringing the food to the mouth, trained classroom staff can provide it. If a child is able to feed himself but not within the time allotted to typical peers, the IEP team should consider how much of a priority self-feeding is among the child's other educational and future transitional needs.

Maintaining and Changing Position. Children in school typically stand, move around and sit on floors and seats in classrooms, lunchrooms, busses, bathrooms and other environments. School activities can range from sitting quietly for an hour to moving every few minutes. For some children, sitting for long periods is a challenge to posture and stability, as well as attention. For others, moving from place to place takes maximum effort. Maintaining and changing positions are necessary for physical health and well being, but also enable children to participate in necessary and preferred occupations. Some children with disabilities must rely on adults to move them and secure them safely. Therapy interventions address emerging mobility needs of children that have an impact on safe engagement and participation in the school environment. (AOTA 2008) These situations may include sitting in standard or adapted seating during classroom instruction or writing assignments, sitting on the floor and getting up, moving from a wheelchair to another chair or toilet, or boarding, traveling in, and disembarking from a vehicle. (Coster et al., 1998) OTs collaborate with other school staff to ensure stability and mobility that is

If a child has IEP goals related to eating, it is likely that a number of people, including a school OT, are involved in the development of strategies related to a child's eating needs in school.

A report from a swallow study or clearance from a physician based on a swallow study is the most definitive information related to safe oral feeding.

appropriate to the child's needs. These skills and accommodations provide the foundation for community mobility, recreational movement, and the ability to use and control objects in the environment.

Children with disabilities may have special securing or positioning needs in school or in vehicles. These physical modifications are provided only to maintain orthopedic, medical, or ergonomic positions. They are never used as a restraint to control the child's behavior in school environments. (Wisconsin Department of Public Instruction, 2009) Chapter 7 describes wheelchair and vehicle mobility in more detail.

Behavior regulation. Positive Behavioral Intervention and Supports (PBIS) is a systemic approach to proactive, school-wide behavior based on a Response to Intervention (RtI) model. (Wisconsin Department of Public Instruction 2010b) It is mentioned earlier in the chapter under *Functional Behavioral Assessment.* PBIS apply evidence-based programs, practices and strategies for all students to increase academic performance, improve safety, decrease problem behavior, and establish a positive school culture. The PBIS model has resulted in dramatic reductions in disciplinary interventions and increases in academic achievement. PBIS applies a team-based, problem-solving process that considers systems, data, practices, and outcomes.

- Systems refer to the policies, procedures, and decision-making processes that consider school-wide, classroom, and individual student systems. Systems support accurate and durable implementation of practices and use data-based decision-making.

- Data are used to guide decision-making processes and measure outcomes. Data support the selection and evaluation of practices and systems.

- Practices include the strategies and programs that are used to directly enhance student learning outcomes and teacher instructional approaches.

- Outcomes are academic and behavioral targets that are endorsed and emphasized by students, families and educators and are measured using the gathered data. (Wisconsin Department of Public Instruction 2009)

Following school rules, resolving ordinary peer conflicts, making and keeping friends, coping with frustration and anger, problem solving, and understanding social etiquette are examples of social competence. Social competence refers to having the social, emotional, and cognitive skills to be able to participate in the many different relationships in a person's everyday life. (AOTA, 2008) School OTs collaborate with other school staff to

- enable the child to develop social and cognitive skills through playground skill groups, social-emotional learning activities, social stories, explorations of the role of friend, and activities that help a child adapt to unalterable aspects of his or her disability.

- help the child learn to regulate overactive or underactive sensory systems.

- help the child incorporate sensory and movement activities to support attention and learning.

- break down learning tasks and homework routines.

- organize supplies and the environment to improve attention and decrease the effect of sensory overload.

Sensory integration is a term that is often used by OTs in relation to behavioral self-regulation. It describes a normal part of human development and ongoing daily life. It refers to the neurological process of receiving information from any of the senses and organizing it for use. The term *sensory integration* can be used to describe

- a general process that occurs naturally in most children and matures through typical childhood activities.

- a specific theory of learning and behavior developed by A. Jean Ayres, Ph.D., author of *Sensory Integration and Learning Disorders*.

- a specific set of occupational therapy treatment activities.

The senses described in sensory integration theory by Ayres and others are

- visual and auditory, the far or distal senses most frequently used in classroom learning.

- tactile and proprioceptive, the near or proximal senses of touch and body movement involved in kinesthetic learning.

- vestibular, the sense of head movement and head position that is closely related to vision, hearing and other neurological processes .

- olfactory and gustatory, the senses of smell and taste, which are closely related to alertness and emotion. (Ayres 1972; Fisher, et al. 1991)

A fundamental assumption of sensory integration theory is that learning is based on the ability to filter, integrate, and respond to sensory information. The efficiency of sensory integration varies from child to child. When a child has severely inefficient sensory integration, the child's interaction with people, places, objects, or events in the educational environment is likely to be impaired. A child with any disability may have impaired sensory integration. This is sometimes called sensory integration dysfunction, or sensory processing disorder.

School OTs have various levels of training in sensory integration theory and intervention. It is not necessary for an OT to have a specialized certification in sensory integration test administration to be able to assess children with impaired sensory integration or sensory processing disorder (SPD). Many OTs do find such training beneficial. Intervention focused on prevention or compensation involves modification of the environment or the child's routines, as well as collaboration with the child's teachers and parents. AOTA recognizes sensory integration as one of several theories and methods used by OTs and OTAs working with children in school towards the desired outcome of health and

Sensory integration is a term that is often used by OTs in relation to behavioral self-regulation. It refers to the neurological process of receiving information from any of the senses and organizing it for use.

participation through engagement in occupations that allow participation in a child's daily life. (AOTA 2008) A growing body of research supports a link between sensory processing disorders and childhood coping skills, such as handling new situations, shifting plans, controlling impulses and activity level, using self-protecting behaviors, applying learning to new situations and balancing independence with dependence on others. (May-Benson 2000) These are functional skills in which the effectiveness of intervention may be measured by goal attainment scaling or other progress monitoring.

Movement and exercise are also important components in self-regulation, mental health and cognitive learning. Aerobic activity has been shown to be as effective as psychotropic medication in balancing the effects of stress hormones in many individuals. (Ratey 2008) OTs collaborate with physical education teachers, classroom teachers and PTs to ensure that children with disabilities have movement experiences that support their health and learning.

A growing body of research supports a link between sensory processing disorders and childhood coping skills.

In the past ten years, interest in the use of sensory modalities to improve coping strategies of individuals with behavioral challenges began to increase. Inpatient mental health units across the nation became actively involved in seclusion and restraint reduction programs (Champagne and Stromberg 2004; Leadholm 2007) Controversy surrounds the use of seclusion and physical restraint in school-based programs, and use of these interventions carries a high degree of risk for being misunderstood. Both techniques are used only as a last resort in cases of danger to the student or others. (DPI, 2009) Like mental health units, schools have sometimes developed sensory rooms to provide environments and activities that are conducive to positive responses and a decrease in the student's sense of distress. Sensory rooms are quite different from seclusion rooms. They are used as a preventive measure and furnished with the sensory needs and limitations of particular children in mind. OTs usually regulate and often supervise the child's initial interactions with the specially designed environment. When they develop and use sensory rooms and sensory modalities, school personnel should adhere to the guidance in Chapter 7 related to safe use of equipment by trained personnel, documentation of equipment use, and maintenance of equipment.

Adaptations. A school OT may be involved in providing an assistive technology service. A complete discussion of assistive technology is in chapter 7. Assistive technology includes devices that range from low to high in technical complexity. Usually referred to as *accommodations*, they are part of changes to the environment that provide students with an opportunity to be successful and demonstrate what they know or have learned. Accommodations do not change the standard or the expectations of the student compared to nondisabled peers. As such, they may be provided to students as part of standardized testing and described on the student's IEP. They may also be provided as part of the student's daily education, and described on the student's IEP as supplementary aids and services. These may include architectural or transportation accommodations, as well as accommodations for behavior, cognition, communication, activities of daily living, and classroom work. Other types of adaptations may be called *modifications*. Modifications do change curricular or behavioral expectations, or standards for individual students. These may be described on the student's IEP as program modifications.

Task Behavior and Completion. Some of the activities required of children in school include listening and watching with attention, initiating and completing assignments, finding and storing materials, recording information, studying, and asking for help. (Coster et al. 1998) Children with disabilities may have performance skills and patterns that do not match the demands of school activities and environments. This mismatch may make it difficult for a child to organize and complete required tasks. OTs collaborate with other school staff to assess the purpose of a task; task demands such as objects, space and time required to complete the task; the roles and expectations of others involved in the task; and the discrepancies between the way a specific child performs the task and the way most other children perform the task. (Griswold 1994; Rainforth and York-Barr, 1997) Compensatory strategies are specific to the activity, context, and student. They include

- teaching the child alternative strategies for accomplishing the task.

- changing the amount of time allotted to the task (altering the activity or the activity demands).

- structuring the spatial nature of the task (adapting the context or environment in which the child performs).

- adapting objects used (improving the child's performance through assistive devices).

- eliminating the task entirely.

Functional communication, socialization, play. Play or leisure is another primary occupational performance area in occupational therapy. Among young children in school, play is an important means of exploring the environment, interacting with others, and developing sensory motor skills. As children get older, social interaction skills and a sense of self continue to develop through play and leisure skills. OTs collaborate with other educators to assess components of a child's play and leisure activities in early childhood classrooms, in physical education classes, during extracurricular activities, and at recess. Therapists and educators may provide intervention that has an impact on play and leisure skills or use play to improve other performance areas. Examples of occupational therapy intervention include

- adapting toys for a young child who has difficulty using her hands.

- collaborating with a physical education teacher to design activities for a child who has a low tolerance for touch and movement.

- teaming with a special education teacher to help adolescents explore adult leisure activities and modify them for successful performance.

OTs collaborate with other school staff to assess the purpose of a task, task demands, the roles and expectations of others involved in the task, and the discrepancies between the way a specific child performs the task and the way most other children perform the task.

Hygiene and personal care awareness, and safety. Activities of daily living (ADL) are a primary performance area in occupational therapy. Children perform ADL in school when toileting, washing hands, and engaging in other personal care activities. Youth learn more advanced independent living skills and instrumental activities of daily living as they prepare for adult life. Teachers and paraprofessionals are usually the persons who supervise ADL in school, and special education teachers often teach ADL. OTs work with teachers to assess functional abilities and deficits in ADL and related performance components. Occupational therapy intervention frequently involves collaborative service to those who are with the child on a daily basis, and the use of compensatory strategies. Direct services may also be required when children are developing performance components or need specialized strategies.

Transition. Transition services are the coordinated set of activities that help prepare a student for life after high school graduation. In Wisconsin, students who are fourteen years of age or older within the timeframe of their current IEPs must have transition requirements addressed in their IEPs. The transition requirements include having measurable postsecondary goals based on age-appropriate transition assessments related to training, education, employment and, where appropriate, independent living skills. A description of transition services, including courses of study, needed to assist the students in reaching the goals is also required. In addition to the areas of intervention described in the previous pages, school OTs address activities that are unique to youth with disabilities in school. They include job analysis, functional capacity evaluation, independent living skills assessment and training, and driving assessment and modifications.

The definition of Activity Demands in the *Framework* illustrates how OTs are skilled in conducting activity analysis for job requirements and internships in both school programs and community-based partnerships. (AOTA 2008) When OTs assess activity demands, they consider the

- tools, materials, and equipment used in the process of carrying out the activity.

- physical environmental requirements of the activity (size, arrangement, surface, lighting, temperature, noise, humidity, ventilation).

- social structure and demands that may be required by the activity.

- process used to carry out the activity (specific steps, sequence, timing requirements).

- usual skills that would be required by any performer to carry out the activity.

- physiological functions of body systems required to support the actions used to perform the activity.

- anatomical parts that are required to perform the activity.

OTs complement the assessment of job requirements by performing a functional capacity evaluation (FCE) of the student. This is a physical assessment of an individual's ability to perform a work-related activity. An FCE usually consists of medical record review, musculoskeletal screening and physical ability testing.

Physical ability testing may include graded strength activities such as lifting, carrying, pushing and pulling; position tolerance activities such as standing, sitting, and stooping; and mobility activities such as walking, crawling, and climbing. An FCE may also include information about an individual's dexterity, coordination, balance, endurance, and other job-specific testing. The FCE report typically includes an overall level of work, a summary of physical abilities in the language used by the U.S. Department of Labor (2011), information about consistency of effort, job match information, and recommendations. (Page et al. 2007)

A third area of transition where OTs provide service is independent living. School OTs may conduct transition assessments of life skills that promote independent living. They may also participate in curriculum development and instruction of life skills. The *Framework* (AOTA 2008) divides independent living skills into activities of daily living (ADL) and instrumental activities of daily living (IADL) ADL are oriented toward taking care of one's own body and include:

School OTs may conduct transition assessments of life skills that promote independent living.

- Bathing

- Showering

- Bowel and bladder management

- Dressing

- Eating

- Feeding

- Functional mobility

- Personal device care

- Personal hygiene and grooming

- Sexual activity

- Sleep and rest

- Toilet hygiene

IADL are oriented toward interacting with the environment and are often complex and generally optional in nature, in that they may be delegated to another. IADL include:

- Care of others (including selecting and supervising caregivers)

- Care of pets

- Child rearing

- Communication device use

- Community mobility

- Financial management

- Health management and maintenance

- Home establishment and management

- Meal preparation and cleanup

- Safety procedures and emergency responses

- Shopping

Community mobility is defined by the *Framework* as "moving around in the community and using public or private transportation, such as driving, walking, bicycling, or accessing and riding in buses, taxi cabs, or other public transportation systems." (AOTA 2008) The assessment of transportation needs has an impact on a student's access to employment, housing, social, educational, and recreational opportunities. (AOTA 2008) For youth in transition, driving is an age-appropriate activity that is often of great interest. A school district that offers driver education to the general student population must also offer it to students with disabilities who have the capacity to drive. (Thiel, 2005) Students with disabilities may encounter barriers to driving in the areas of executive function, visual, sensory or motor skills. When the IEP team considers a student's potential for learning to drive, the school OT may provide a pre-driving screening. The OT can identify potential barriers and recommend interventions prior to a formal driving evaluation by a driving rehabilitation specialist.

When the IEP team considers a student's potential for learning to drive, the school OT may provide a pre-driving screening.

Record Keeping

School OTs should keep regular, ongoing documentation of each child's occupational therapy intervention. In addition to evaluation reports and treatment plans, standard documentation for school occupational therapy includes

- attendance records that document the amount and frequency of service the therapist provides to the child.

- progress notes on treatment plans and data collection on responses to intervention.

- notes on contacts with parents.

- notes on contacts with physicians and recommendations.

- notes on contacts with teachers and recommendations.

- discontinuance reports.

These records help the OT focus on educationally relevant intervention as well as provide helpful background and historical treatment information when a child transfers from one therapist to another. Records form a basis for the OT to assess the quality of the occupational therapy service, as well as determine typical amounts of therapy needed to accomplish similar outcomes with other children. Medicaid and other medical insurance providers may require OTs to keep other specific records to obtain third-party payment for occupational therapy.

Ethics

AOTA revised the Occupational Therapy Code of Ethics in 2010. The Code of Ethics is a public statement of principles used to promote and maintain high standards of conduct within the profession. Members of AOTA are committed to promoting inclusion, diversity, independence, and safety for all recipients in various stages of life, health, and illness and to empower all beneficiaries of occupational therapy. This commitment extends beyond service recipients to include professional colleagues, students, educators, businesses, and the community. The specific purpose of the AOTA Occupational Therapy Code of Ethics is to

- Identify and describe the principles supported by the occupational therapy profession.

- Educate the general public and members regarding established principles to which occupational therapy personnel are accountable.

- Socialize occupational therapy personnel new to the practice to expected standards of conduct.

- Assist occupational therapy personnel in recognition and resolution of ethical dilemmas. (AOTA 2010)

Appendix D contains a link to the Occupational Therapy Code of Ethics.

Members of AOTA are committed to promoting inclusion, diversity, independence, and safety for all recipients in various stages of life, health, and illness.

References

American Occupational Therapy Association (AOTA). 1994. "Uniform Terminology for Occupational Therapy Third Edition." *American Journal of Occupational Therapy* 48: 1047-1059.

___. 1995. "Occupation." *American Journal of Occupational Therapy* 49: 1015-18.

___. 2002. "Occupational Therapy Practice Framework: Domain and Process." *American Journal of Occupational Therapy* 56: 609-39.

___. 2008. "Occupational Therapy Practice Framework: Domain and Process Second Edition." *American Journal of Occupational Therapy* 62: 25-683. http://www.aota.org/Practitioners/Official/Guidelines/41089.aspx (accessed August 2, 2010).

___. 2009. "Specialized Knowledge and Skills in Feeding, Eating, and Swallowing for Occupational Therapy Practice." *American Journal of Occupational Therapy* 61:686-700.

___. 2010. "Standards of Practice for Occupational Therapy." *American Journal of Occupational Therapy* 64: (in press). http://www.aota.org/Practitioners/Official/Standards/36194.aspx (accessed August 2, 2010).

Asher, A.V. 2006. "Handwriting Instruction in Elementary Schools." *American Journal of Occupational Therapy* 60:461-471.

Asher, I.E. 2007. *Occupational Therapy Assessment Tools: An Annotated Index.* 3rd ed. Bethesda, MD: AOTA Press.

Ayres, A.J. 1972. *Sensory Integration and Learning Disorders.* Los Angeles: Western Psychological Services.

Baker, B. 1999. "Principles of Motor Learning For School-Based Occupational Therapy Practitioners." *School System Special Interest Section Quarterly* 6: 1-4.

Baumgart, D., L. Brown, I. Pumpian, J. Nisbet, A. Ford, M. Sweet, R. Messina, and J. Schroeder. 1982. "Principle of Partial Participation and Individualized Adaptations in Educational Programs for Severely Handicapped Students." *Journal of the Association for the Severely Handicapped* 7.2: 17-27.

Carlson, C. 2008. "Mastery Monitoring: Measuring Progress on Multistep Tasks." *OT Practice*, May 12, 2008.

CESA 12. 1999. "Functional Behavior Assessment: A Study Guide." http://www.dpi.wi.gov/sped/doc/fba-study.doc (accessed August 2, 2010).

Champagne, T. and N. Stromberg. 2004. "Sensory Approaches in Inpatient Psychiatric Settings: Innovative Alternatives to Seclusion and Restraint." *Journal of Psychosocial Nursing* 42(9): 35-44.

Chiang, B. and B.J. Rylance. 2000. *Occupational and Physical Therapy Caseload Size: Service Provision and Perceptions of Efficacy.* Oshkosh: University of Wisconsin-Oshkosh.

Clark, G.F. 1992. "Oral-Motor and Feeding Issues," in *Classroom Applications for School-Based Practice.* Ed. C.B. Royeen. Rockville, MD: American Occupational Therapy Association.

Cohn, E. 2001. "Parent Perspectives of Occupational Therapy Using a Sensory Integration Approach." *American Journal of Occupational Therapy* 55: 285-294.

Cope, S.M. 2005. Presentation at Statewide School-Based OT/PT Conference, October 28, 2005.

Coster, W., T. Deeney, J. Haltiwanger, and S. Haley. 1998. *School Function Assessment.*. San Antonio, TX: Pearson.

Cronbach, L. 1990. *Essentials of Psychological Testing.* 2nd edition. New York: HarperCollins.

Deno. S. 2009. "Ongoing Student Assessment. " RTI Action Network. http://www.rtinetwork.org/essential/assessment/ongoingassessment (accessed August 2, 2010).

Dohrn, E., P. Volpiansky, T. Kratochwill and L. Sanetti. 2006. *Progress Monitoring Toolkit.* Madison: Wisconsin Department of Public Instruction.

Dunn, W. 1990. "A Comparison of Service Provision Models in School-Based Occupational Therapy Services." *Occupational Therapy Journal of Research* 10.5: 300-320.

___. 1991. "Consultation as a Process: How, When, and Why?" In *School-Based Practice for Related Services,* ed. C.B. Royeen. Rockville, MD: American Occupational Therapy Association.

Dunn, W., and K. Westman. 1995. "Current Knowledge That Affects School-Based Practice and an Agenda for Action." *School System Special Interest Section Newsletter* 2.1: 1-2.

Dysart, A., and G. Tomlin. 2002. "Factors Related to Evidence-Based Practice among U.S. Occupational Therapy Clinicians." *American Journal of Occupational Therapy* 56, 275-284.

Fisher, A., E. Murray, and A. Bundy. 1991. *Sensory Integration: Theory and Practice.* Philadelphia: F.A. Davis Company.

Flood, L., J. Johnson, T. Prill. 2001. "Targeting Handwriting." Unpublished action research report, Edgerton School District, Edgerton, Wisconsin.

Giangreco, M.F. 1986. "Effects of Integrated Therapy: A Pilot Study." *Journal of the Association for Persons with Severe Handicaps* 11: 205-08.

Griswold, L.A. 1994. "Ethnographic Analysis: A Study of Classroom Environments." *American Journal of Occupational Therapy* 48.5: 397-402.

Hanft, B. & J. Shepard. 2008. *Collaborating for Student Success: A Guide for School-Based Occupational Therapy.* Bethesda, MD: AOTA Press.

Holm, M. 2000. "Our Mandate for the New Millennium: Evidence-Based Practice." *American Journal of Occupational Therapy* 54, 575-585.

Kiresuk, T., and R. Sherman. 1968. "Goal Attainment Scaling: A General Method Of Evaluating Comprehensive Mental Health Programs." *Community Mental Health Journal,* 4:443-53.

Knippenberg, C and B. Hanft. 2004. "The Key to Educational Relevance: Occupation throughout the School Day." *School System Special Interest Section Quarterly,* Volume 11(4).

Law, M. and C. Baum. 1998. "Evidence-based Occupational Therapy." *Canadian Journal of Occupational Therapy* 65(3): 131-135.

Mailloux, Z., T.A. May-Benson, C.A. Summers, L.J. Miller, B., Brett-Green, J.P. Burke, E.S. Cohn, J.A. Koomar, L.D. Parham, S.S. Roley, R.C. Schaaf, and S.A. Schoen. 2007. "Goal Attainment Scaling As a Measure of Meaningful Outcomes for Children with Sensory Integration Disorders." *American Journal of Occupational Therapy,* 61: 254-59.

May-Benson, T. 2000. "'I Can't Do It...!' Examining Coping Skills in Children with SI Dysfunction." *OT Practice Online.* http://www.aota.org/Pubs/OTP/1997-2007/Features/2000/37123.aspx (accessed August 2, 2010).

McGregor, G., and R. Vogelsberg. 1998. *Inclusive Schooling Practices: Pedagogical and Research Foundations.* Baltimore: Brookes.

McWilliam, R. and B .Clingenpeel. 2003. "Functional Intervention Planning: The Routines-Based Interview." Vanderbilt University: National Individualizing Preschool Inclusion Project.

McWilliam, R. and S. Scott. 2003. "Integrating Therapy into the Classroom." Vanderbilt University: National Individualizing Preschool Inclusion Project.

Moyers, P. and L. Dale. 2007. *The Guide to Occupational Therapy Practice.* 2nd ed. Bethesda, MD: AOTA Press.

National Center on Student Progress Monitoring. 2010. http://www.studentprogress.org / (accessed August 2, 2010).

Ottenbacher, K.J. and A. Cusick. 1990. "Goal Attainment Scaling as a Method of Clinical Service Evaluation." *American Journal of Occupational Therapy* 44: 519-525.

Page, J., J. Clinger, M. Dodson, and K. Maltchev. 2007. "Functional Capacity Evaluation." AOTA Work Programs SIS Fact Sheet. http://www.aota.org/Practitioners/PracticeAreas/Work/Fact-Sheets/35117.aspx (accessed August 2, 2010).

Rainforth, B., and J. York-Barr. 1997. *Collaborative Teams for Students with Severe Disabilities.* 2nd ed. Baltimore: Paul H. Brookes.

Ratey, J. 2008. *Spark: The Revolutionary New Science of Exercise and the Brain.* New York: Little, Brown and Company.

Rea, P., V. McLaughlin, and C. Walther-Thomas. 2002. "Outcomes for Students with Disabilities in Inclusive and Pullout Programs." *Exceptional Children 68*: 203-222.

Sackett, D.L, W.S. Richardson, W.M.C. Rosenberg, and R.B. Haynes. 2000. *Evidence-based Medicine: How to Practice and Teach EBM.* 2nd Edition. London: Churchill-Livingstone.

Sarracino, T. (2002). Using Evidence to Inform School-Based Practice. *School System Special Interest Section Quarterly*, 9, 1-4.

Silverman, M.K., K.F. Stratman, and R.O. Smith. 2000. "Measuring Assistive Technology Outcomes in Schools Using Functional Assessment." *Diagnostique,* 25(4):307-25.

Swinth, Y., K.C. Spencer, and L.L. Jackson. 2007. *Occupational Therapy: Effective School-Based Practices within a Policy Context.* (COPSSE Document Number OP-3). Gainesville, FL: University of Florida, Center on Personnel Studies in Special Education.

Thiel, Randall. 2005. "Driving with a Disability." Wisconsin Assistive Technology Initiative, Wisconsin Department of Public Instruction. May 2005.

U.S. Department of Labor. 2011. *O*NET Resource Center.* http://www.onetcenter.org (accessed May 2, 2011).

Wisconsin Department of Public Instruction. 2009. "DPI Directives for the Appropriate Use of Seclusion and Physical Restraint in Special Education Programs." http://www.dpi.wi.gov/sped/doc/secrestrgd.doc (accessed August 2, 2010).

___. 2010. "Wisconsin Model Academic Standards." http://www.dpi.wi.gov/standards/index.html (accessed August 2, 2010).

World Health Organization. "International Classification of Functioning, Disability and Health, ICF." http://www.who.int/classifications/icf/en/ (accessed March 9, 2010)

Other Resources

American Occupational Therapy Association (AOTA). 2003. "Applying Sensory Integration Framework in Educationally Related Occupational Therapy Practice." *American Journal of Occupational Therapy* 57:652-59.

Bar-Lev, N., P. Bober, G. Dietz, C. Salzer, S. Endress, and E. Weiman. 2007. *Special Education in Plain Language: A User-friendly Interactive Handbook on Special Education Laws, Policies and Practices in Wisconsin, Third Edition.* Madison, WI: Wisconsin Department of Public Instruction. http://www.specialed.us/pl-07/pl07-index.html (accessed August 2, 2010).

Bober, P. 2002. "Moving Toward Evidence-Based Practice in Schools: Wisconsin's Model." *School System Special Interest Quarterly*, 9 (4): 1-3, 6.

Leadholm, B. 2007. "Seclusion and Restraint Philosophy Statement. "Commonwealth of Massachusetts Department of Mental Health. http://www.mass.gov/Eeohhs2/docs/dmh/rsri/sr_philosophy_statement_9_2007.pdf (accessed August 2, 2010).

Telzrow, C. F., and J.J. Beebe. 2002. "Best Practices in Facilitating Intervention Adherence and Integrity," in A. Thomas & J. Grimes (Eds.), *Best Practices in School Psychology IV:* 503-16. Bethesda, MD: National Association of School Psychologists.

University of Oklahoma Health Sciences Center. 2007. "School Outcomes Measure Administrative Guide."

Department Of Rehabilitation Science, P.O. Box 26901, Oklahoma City, OK 73190-1090. http://www.ah.ouhsc.edu/somresearch/adminGuide.pdf (accessed August 2, 2010).

Wisconsin Department of Public Instruction. 2010. "Positive Behavioral Intervention and Supports (PBIS)." http://www.dpi.wi.gov/rti/pbis.html (accessed August 2, 2010).

School-Based Physical Therapy

5

Physical therapists (PTs) in school-based practice discover that working in schools requires knowledge of pediatric physical therapy; collaboration with other team members including parents, educators, and staff; and provision of interventions that help students perform functional tasks at school. A unique challenge for school-based PTs is providing services to students in accordance with special education law and within the context of the practice of physical therapy.

Competencies for School-Based PTs

The American Physical Therapy Association (APTA) Section on Pediatrics identifies nine competency content areas for PTs working in schools. These competencies give an overview of the roles and responsibilities of the school based PT. Figure 19 on pages 98-99 describes the competencies.

Conceptual Frameworks

National health organizations adopt conceptual frameworks to describe the consequence of disease and injury on the person and society. Such organizations include the National Center for Medical Rehabilitation Research (NCMRR), National Institutes of Health, and the World Health Organization. One of the original frameworks is the disablement model, also known as the Nagi model or NCMRR model. The APTA applies this model in the *Guide to Physical Therapist Practice (APTA 1999),* its standard publication and a main resource for this chapter.

Disablement Model
The basic concepts of the disablement model are that pathology leads to impairment which may result in functional limitations and cause disability. The list below describes disablement model terminology.

Pathology refers to the conditions of the disease or the disease process. An example is the decrease in the muscle protein dystropin in children with muscular dystrophy.

Impairment refers to the loss or abnormality of physiological, psychological, or anatomical function. An example is decreased muscle strength or balance problems.

Functional Limitation refers to the restriction of the ability to perform a physical action, activity, or task in an efficient, typically expected, or competent manner. Examples include the inability to put on a coat, walk up bus steps, or walk down a hallway.

A unique challenge for school-based PTs is providing services to students in accordance with special education law and within the context of the practice of physical therapy.

Figure 19 Competencies for School-Based Physical Therapists

Competency Area 1: Context of Therapy Practice in Education Settings

- Know the structure, global goals, and responsibilities of the public education system including special education.

- Know federal, state, and local laws and regulations that affect the delivery of services to students with disabilities.

- Know theoretical and functional orientation of a variety of professionals serving students within the educational system.

- Assist students in accessing community organizations, resources and activities.

Competency Area 2: Wellness and Prevention in Schools

- Implement school-wide screening program with school nurses, physical education teachers, and teachers.

- Promote child safety and wellness using knowledge of environmental safety measures.

Competency Area 3: Team Collaboration

- Form partnerships and work collaboratively with other team members, especially teachers, to promote an effective plan of care.

- Function as a consultant.

- Educate school personnel and family to promote the inclusion of students within the educational experience.

- Supervise personnel and professional students.

Competency Area 4: Examination and Evaluation in Schools

- Identify strengths and needs of students.

- Collaboratively determine examination and evaluation process.

- Determine students' ability to participate in meaningful school activities.

- Utilize valid, reliable, cost-effective, and nondiscriminatory evaluation instruments.

Competency Area 5: Planning

- Actively participate in the development of IEPs.

Competency Area 6: Intervention

- Adapt environment to facilitate access to and participation in student activities.

- Use various types and methods of service provision for individualized student interventions.

- Promote skill acquisition, fluency, and generalization to enhance overall development, learning, and student participation.

- Imbed therapy intervention into the context of student activities and routines.

Competency Area 7: Documentation

- Produce useful written documentation.

- Collaboratively monitor and modify IEPs.

- Evaluate and document the effectiveness of therapy programs.

Competency Area 8: Administrative Issues in Schools

- Demonstrate flexibility, priority setting, and effective time management strategies.

- Obtain resources and data necessary to justify establishing a new therapy program or altering an existing program.

- Serve as a leader.

- Serve as a manager.

Competency Area 9: Research

- Demonstrate knowledge of current research relating to child development, medical care, educational practices, and implications for therapy.

- Apply knowledge of research to the selection of therapy intervention strategies, service delivery systems, and therapeutic procedures.

- Partake in program evaluation and clinical research activities with the appropriate supervision.

Effgen, Chiarello, and Milbourne, 2007, 266-74. Adapted with permission from Wolters Kluwer Health, Lippincott Williams and Wilkins.

Disability is the inability to engage in age-specific, gender-related roles in a particular social context and physical environment such as student, athlete, or worker. Disability occurs when there is a discrepancy between the child's performance and the demands of the environment. An example is the inability of a student to move around the classroom to participate in class activities.

Handicap is a societal limitation. An example is the inability of a student to use the library because it is not accessible by wheelchair.

Guide to Physical Therapist Practice

The APTA's *Guide to Physical Therapist Practice* describes accepted PT practice, standardizes terminology, and delineates preferred practice patterns. The disablement model is the conceptual basis for the *Guide to Physical Therapist Practice*, so understanding disablement allows professionals to understand and organize physical therapy practice. The *Guide to Physical Therapist Practice* describes and emphasizes the role of prevention and wellness strategies in optimizing function. Familiarity with the *Guide to Physical Therapist Practice* is important as the concepts and terminology in the *Guide to Physical Therapist Practice* also appear in the Physical Therapy Practice Act, the state statute that governs physical therapy practice in all settings including schools. (Chapter 448.50, Wis. Stats.)

The *Guide to Physical Therapist Practice* states that the PT alleviates or prevents impairment, functional limitation, and disability. Through patient/client management, the PT determines the interrelationships among the severity of impairment, extent of functional limitation, and degree of disability. Impairment may lead to loss of function and loss of function may lead to disability. However, one does not always lead to the next. Impairment does not always result in the inability to perform a task. Likewise, limited function does not necessarily prevent performance of a specific role. Remediation of impairments is not the outcome or goal of physical therapy intervention. The PT only addresses impairments as they relate to functional outcomes, disability, or secondary prevention. For example, a PT works with two students. Both have leg muscular weakness, which is a limitation at the impairment level. The first student moves independently around the school with crutches, but is unable to manage the school bus steps. Through evaluation, the PT determines the student's leg weakness interferes with the ability to manage the bus steps. The PT would intervene at the impairment level and work with this student on leg strengthening exercises to enable the student to manage the bus steps, a functional activity. In contrast, the second student moves independently throughout the school building with a regular wheelchair, but is unable to maneuver on the exterior school grounds. The PT would not work with the second student on leg strengthening exercises. Instead the PT would work with this student only at the functional activity level and would develop sessions for the student to practice wheelchair mobility on uneven surfaces, ramps, and curbs.

The *Guide to Physical Therapist Practice* defines the five elements of patient/client management: examination, evaluation, diagnosis, prognosis, intervention, and outcome.

The PT determines the interrelationships among the severity of impairment, extent of functional limitation, and degree of disability.

- *Examination* includes data gathering through patient history, relevant systems reviews, and tests and measures.

- *Evaluation* is the process in which the PT makes clinical judgments based on gathered data.

- *Diagnosis* is the organization of the information into categories or clusters to help determine interventions.

- *Prognosis* is the determination of the level of expected improvement through intervention and the amount of service required.

- *Intervention* is the use of physical therapy methods and techniques.

- *Outcome* is the result of intervention in alleviating or preventing the patient's functional limitations and disability.

The *Guide to Physical Therapist Practice* describes the types of tests and measures that PTs use and the interventions they provide. The *Guide to Physical Therapist Practice* also identifies preferred practice patterns for four categories of conditions: musculoskeletal, neuromuscular, cardiopulmonary, and integumentary (related to the skin.) The practice patterns describe common sets of strategies that PTs use for selected patient diagnostic groups. These practice patterns identify the range of current care options.

Disablement models, described earlier, have evolved into the enablement model.

The basic disablement models, described earlier, have evolved into the current International Classification of Functioning, Disability, and Health (ICF), also referred to as the enablement model. ICF provides an internationally accepted framework for the description of human functioning and disability and describes the complex interaction between health, the environment, and personal factors. Although its Guide *to Physical Therapist Practice* currently uses the disablement model, the APTA in June 2008 joined other world and national health organizations in endorsing the ICF model. APTA will now incorporate ICF language into all its publications, documents, and communications through existing planned review and revision.

International Classification of Functioning, Disability, and Health (ICF)
The ICF provides a description of how a person with a health condition functions in daily life. ICF is a member of the World Health Organization (WHO) Family of International Classifications. ICF is a classification of health and health-related domains that describe body functions and structures, activities, and participation. (WHO 2002) The domains are classified from body, individual and societal perspectives. ICF emphasizes function, health, and participation rather than disease. Since an individual's functioning and disability occurs in a context, ICF also includes a list of environmental and personal factors. The following is a list of ICF terms and their definitions.

- *Body Functions* are physiological functions of body systems.

- *Body Structures* are anatomical parts of the body such as organs, limbs, and their components.

- *Impairments* are problems in body function or structure.

- *Activity* is the execution of a task or action by the individual.

- *Participation* is involvement in a life situation.

- *Environmental Factors* make up the physical, social, and attitudinal environment in which people conduct their lives.

ICF emphasizes a person's functional ability to perform activities and tasks and participate in life. This parallels IDEA requirements that emphasize a student's functional performance as well as participation in the classroom, general curriculum, and grade-level assessments. PTs focus their interventions at the activity and participation levels to allow the student to participate in classroom routines and school activities. At the impairment level, the PT sometimes works with a student on a dimension of movement such as flexibility, strength, accuracy, speed, adaptability, or endurance (Allen, 2007) only when the impairment interferes with the student's function or participation at school. The ICF model also indicates that activities and participation can influence impairments and pathology. This aspect of the model allows PTs to intervene to prevent impairments. For example, a child who uses a wheelchair may develop pressure sores. A therapist can use the model preventatively to design a positioning program to stop the development of pressure sores.

Medical Referral and Medical Information

A medical referral is not required when evaluating or serving a child with a disability under IDEA. A medical referral is also not required for other students, such as those with a 504 plan.

A medical referral is not required when evaluating or serving a child with a disability under IDEA. A medical referral is also not required for other students, such as those with a 504 plan, when services meet the requirements in Chapter PT 6.01, Wis. Admin Code. This state law declares that a written referral is not required to provide services related to educational environments for conditioning, injury prevention, and application of biomechanics, treatment of musculoskeletal injuries *except* acute fractures, or soft tissue avulsions (the tearing of skin or other soft tissue). For provision of other services, the PT needs a written referral from a physician, chiropractor, dentist, podiatrist or advanced practice nurse prescriber.

Although it is the district's responsibility to provide physical therapy, the district may bill the child's Medicaid under School-Based Services (SBS) or other medical insurance under certain circumstances. If the school district has a *Request for a Waiver to Wisconsin Medicaid Prescription Requirements Under the School-Based Services Benefit* form on file with Wisconsin Medicaid, a prescription is only required under limited circumstances. Chapter 8 includes a link to the Medicaid waiver form.

The PT may evaluate a child without medical information; but before providing services, the PT must have medical information from a licensed physician. Most students have current medical information which parents share with the district. For a transfer student, medical information from a licensed physician in the state of origin or other Wisconsin community may be available. Some students may come to school with little or no medical information. Children who are homeless or who are displaced due to natural disasters enroll in school and may bring transfer records or have no medical records. Existing data in the child's transfer records, out-of-state IEPs, or other pupil records may include information from a licensed physician. When this information is unavailable, an examination by a licensed physician is required. The district must ensure it is obtained at no cost to the parent.

The PT uses professional judgment to determine what, and how much information is needed in order to provide safe and appropriate services to the child, and this may vary considerably from child to child. For example, when a child's medical condition is stable or uncomplicated, as is true of some children with specific learning disabilities, the therapist may need to check periodically with the parents to see if new medical information is available. However, if the child experiences significant changes due to degenerative processes or surgical intervention, the therapist will require current medical information. The therapist must know about possible contraindications to interventions as well as the child's current status.

The PT uses professional judgment to determine what, and how much information is needed in order to provide safe and appropriate services to the child.

If the therapist needs to contact the physician directly, the therapist or other designated school employee must ask the child's parents to sign a consent or release-of-information form. The therapist can contact only the specific agencies or individuals designated on the form and only during the period of time specified on the form. Some districts request that parents sign the release-of-information form at the IEP meeting so the form is available and on file. Schools must treat as confidential the written records health care providers send to the school or the therapists prepare from verbal information given by health care providers. School district employees may have access to those records only if they need them to comply with a requirement in federal or state law or if the child's parent gives informed consent. (Chapter 146, Wis. Stats.)

Occasionally when therapists seek permission for communication with a physician or other health care providers, the parent responds that the child does not have a doctor, the physician responds that he or she has not seen the child recently enough to provide relevant information, or the parent denies access. The therapist should seek assistance from the director of special education to work with the parent to obtain medical information, explaining the district must provide safe and legal therapy. The school district cannot deny related services to a child due to the difficulty in obtaining medical information, so it is helpful to try and work out a solution with the parent. The district may suggest that only pertinent information is released, as the parent may be reluctant to share all medical information. The district may ask for assistance of the parent liaison in communicating with the parent or seek mediation. The district may be required to provide transportation to a doctor's appointment or provide financial assistance for the appointment to the parents. Figure 17 in chapter 4 is a sample medical information worksheet that may clarify the exchange of information between the therapist and physician.

Initial Evaluation and Examination

Initial evaluation in special education corresponds to evaluation and examination in physical therapy. A special education evaluation helps the IEP team answer the following questions.

- What is the child doing in school now?

- What are the child's strengths?

- What are the child's academic needs?

- What is the child's functional performance?

- What are the parents' concerns?

An initial evaluation begins with the review of existing data, which helps the IEP team determine the need for additional tests and avoid unnecessary testing. Existing data may provide information about the student's communication skills, cognitive abilities, and learning styles. As part of the IEP team, the PT reviews this information and decides whether additional data are required. Existing data may provide information about the student's *history* in terms of general health status, pertinent surgical procedures, growth and development, current functional activity level, cultural background, and medication. Existing data may provide *systems review* data regarding the student's general health including cardiopulmonary, musculoskeletal, neuromuscular, and integumentary status. Existing data may also include recent physical therapy assessments, tests, or measures that the school-based PT reviews. Perhaps the student had recently been seen at a multidisciplinary pediatric clinic, and the clinic assessments are available. These tests and measures need not be repeated. As part of the physical therapy evaluation for school-based services, the PT proceeds with *examination,* focusing on the student's functional performance within the school environment. The PT gathers data about the student's ability to perform functional school tasks and to participate in classroom and school activities. The PT considers

- the student's current and anticipated functional expectations.

- the student's current level of participation in educational programs.

- the extent to which the student depends upon help and task modifications to succeed.

- the tasks and skills that limit the student's participation in classroom and school activities.

The PT gathers data about the student's ability to perform functional school tasks and to participate in classroom and school activities.

Tests and Measures

School-based PTs use specific tests and measures to gather data regarding the student's functional performance within the school environment. Pediatric assessment tools may target a particular age group. For students in early childhood (3-5 years), the PT might choose the Functional Independence Measure for Children (WeeFIM) to measure the assistance needed for the child to perform functional activities. The PT may measure the child's level of motor function with the Gross Motor Function Measure (GMFM) or measure the child's functional performance with the Pediatric Evaluation of Disability Inventory (PEDI).

Other assessments are specifically designed for school settings. An example is the School Function Assessment (SFA). The SFA is a standardized criterion-referenced test for children in kindergarten to grade six. The SFA measures a student's performance of functional tasks at school. (Coster et al. 1998) The SFA is divided into three parts.

I. *Participation* examines the student's level of participation in six school settings.

II. *Task Supports* determines the supports currently provided to the student when he or she performs functional tasks.

III. *Activity Performance* looks at the student's ability to initiate and complete specific functional tasks.

The SFA encourages a collaborative approach to assessment because the PT, parent, teacher, occupational therapist (OT), and speech therapist can all contribute to completing the assessment. Or the PT may administer selective SFA scales specific to the difficulty in movement that the student is experiencing. For example, if the student experiences problems moving in the classroom and throughout the school environment, the PT may complete the section on Travel, Maintaining and Changing Positions, Recreational Movement, and Up/Down Stairs.

For older students, the Enderle-Severson Transition Rating Scale (ESTR) is a criterion-referenced assessment of student performance and student future outcomes and goals. (Enderle and Severson 2003) The ESTR provides information about the student's *strengths, needs, preferences, and interests* to assist in transition plans. The PT, as part of the IEP team, works collaboratively with school personnel to complete the scale. This is combined with information from the parent and student to develop the student's transition plan.

Use of Standardized Tests

In the Physical Therapy Practice Act, *testing* means standardized methods or techniques for gathering data. The child is assessed in all areas of suspected disability including motor abilities. When administering a standardized test, the therapist considers its reliability, validity, standard error of measurement, age range covered, and population on which the test was standardized. Any

The SFA encourages a collaborative approach to assessment because the PT, parent, teacher, occupational therapist (OT), and speech therapist can all contribute to completing the assessment.

modifications to the standardized administration of the test require notation. When selecting a test, the therapist considers whether the test is designed to identify delay or whether the test measures change and would monitor progress over time.

More standardized pediatric physical therapy assessment tools are now available. Examples of new functional measures are the Standardized Walking Obstacle Course (SWOC), Timed Up and Go (TUG), Timed Up and Down Stairs Test (TUDS), Pediatric Balance Scale, and the Functional Reach Test (FRT). There are norms for walking 50 feet in elementary school hallways and norms for a six-minute walk test for children. Appendix C provides a list of pediatric physical therapy assessment tools. The list is organized using the ICF model.

"Standardized tests especially those normed against typically developing children often do not help us to identify what the student really needs to access and or participate in the school or community setting. The literature now is supportive of top-down assessments, those tools that help us recognize what the child can do and what he/she needs to do next in order to be successful in school." (Cecere, 2007) PTs may gather and document baseline data for purposes of evaluation, program planning, and progress monitoring by using non-standardized assessments such as ecological inventories or skilled observation.

Functional classification systems provide information for program planning, research, and predicting service needs. Functional classification systems also enhance communication among therapy providers. The expanded Gross Motor Function Classification System (GMFCS-E&R) is based on self-initiated movement, with emphasis on sitting, transfers, and mobility for children with cerebral palsy. Emphasis is on current level of performance in home, school, and community settings. GMFCS distinguishes five levels and each level describes a range of functional abilities and limitations. The general headings for each level are:

I.   walks without limitations

II. walks with limitations

III. walks using a hand-held mobility device

IV. self-mobility with limitations, may use powered mobility

V.   transported in a manual wheelchair

The focus of the GMFCS is on determining the level which best represents the child's present abilities and limitations in gross motor function. Age groups are described for before the second birthday, between the second and fourth birthday, between the fourth and sixth birthday, between the sixth and the twelfth birthday, and between the twelfth and eighteenth birthday. The GMFCS - E&R provides an estimate of a child's future motor capabilities and a prediction of a child's functional status.

The literature now is supportive of top-down assessments, those tools that help us recognize what the child can do and what he/she needs to do next in order to be successful in school.

Another functional classification system is the Manual Ability Classification System (MACS) for children with cerebral palsy, 4 to 18 years. Similar to the GMFCS, the MACS distinguishes five levels of the child's ability to handle objects in daily activities:

I. handles objects easily and successfully

II. handles most objects but with somewhat reduced quality and/or speed of achievement

III. handles objects with difficulty; needs help to prepare and/or modify activities

IV. handles a limited selection of easily managed objects in adapted situations

V. does not handle objects and has severely limited ability to perform even simple actions

Physical Therapy Evaluation

The PT's *evaluation* involves making clinical judgments based on gathered data, which is then shared with the IEP team. The PT considers

- "whether or not clinical finding (impairments, functional limitations, or disabilities) impact on the child's function or participation at school.

- clinical judgment of student's status in relation to needs at school.

- priorities of the student, family and school personnel.

- stability of the condition in relation to function and participation at school.

- chronicity or severity of the current problem.

- developmental expectations in relation to the child's disability and based on most recent research evidence.

- physical environment of the school (e.g. need to negotiate stairs, distances between classes, etc.) in relationship to the student's function.

- strengths and needs of the child in relation to function and participation in the school setting.

- child's progress toward IEP goals." (G. Birmingham, et al. 2006, 24.)

During the IEP team discussion, the PT shares information about the child's strengths, the child's current abilities, and the child's needs for participation in school and classroom activities. This correlates with *diagnosis* in the *Guide to Physical Therapist Practice* as the therapist considers the impact of student's condition on function at school. At the IEP meeting, the PT also shares the determination of the level of improvement that might occur through intervention within the specified time in the IEP. This assists with IEP goal development and correlates with *prognosis* in the *Guide to Physical Therapist Practice*.

Physical Therapy Intervention Plan

The intervention or treatment plan is the framework for implementing the physical therapy required by the child's IEP. PI 11.24 of the Wisconsin Administrative Code requires school PTs to develop physical therapy treatment plans for the child. The IEP sets the direction of physical therapy intervention for a child, and the annual goal states the desired functional outcome. The physical therapy intervention plan includes the following:

- name, birth date, and diagnosis

- precautions

- current functional abilities, movement skills, and physical status

- a restatement of the IEP goals which the therapist will help the child meet

- interventions

- indirect services such as collaboration and coaching

- supervision of assistant, if appropriate

- coordination with outside therapist

- documentation of progress

The PT develops the intervention plan and modifies the plan when indicated.

The PT develops the intervention plan and modifies the plan when indicated. The intervention may be solely used by the therapist who developed it; by a therapist who is substituting for another therapist or receiving a child from another therapist's caseload; or by the PTA who is implementing the intervention developed by the PT. Sample physical therapy intervention plans are included in Appendix B.

Interventions

PTs use various interventions and techniques that encourage functional independence, emphasize student participation in classroom and school activities, and promote fitness and health. Figure 20 on the following page describes common physical therapy interventions.

Figure 20 Physical Therapy Interventions

Type of Physical Therapy Intervention	Examples of Interventions in School-Based Practice
Therapeutic exercise	Balance, coordination, gait, and mobility training; aerobic endurance activities; motor learning; strengthening exercises
Functional training in school activities	Activity performance of motor tasks for travel, maintaining and changing positions, recreational movements, manipulation with movement, using materials, setup and cleanup, eating and drinking, hygiene, clothing management, up and down stair movement, safety
Functional training in self-care	Transfer training from wheelchair to desk, chair, lab stool, floor, or toilet; overuse prevention; orthotic or prosthetic equipment training
Functional training in community	Injury prevention, performance or adaptation of motor tasks related to job training experience (as part of transition)
Prescription, application, and training in use of adaptive equipment	Assistive devices: crutches, canes, walkers, wheelchairs, scooter boards Power devices: motorized wheelchairs and scooters Adaptive devices: seating systems, raised toilet seats, grab bars; supine, prone, or dynamic standers Orthotic devices: braces, shoe inserts, splints Prosthetic limbs Protective devices: cushions, helmets Supportive devices: compression garments, collars, taping
Respiratory and rib cage exercises	Breathing strategies, positioning, movement, and exercises to improve function
Manual therapy	Hands-on techniques for joint and soft tissue mobilization

Physical Agents and Electrotherapeutic Modalities

In clinical and hospital settings, PTs use physical agents (paraffin baths, hot packs, cold packs, whirlpool, and ultrasound) and electrotherapeutic modalities (functional electrical stimulation, neuromuscular electrical stimulation, and biofeedback). Schools generally do not maintain such equipment. School physical therapy often occurs in a classroom setting, and a separate clinical area for providing these interventions seldom exists. The safe use of these modalities in the school environment, their maintenance, and storage also are reasons for not using these interventions in the school setting. For these reasons, school PTs use a variety of interventions other than physical agents and electrotherapeutic modalities to meet treatment or intervention goals. For example, instead of using neuromuscular electrical stimulation to improve ambulation, the school PT develops balance and coordination activities, uses strengthening exercises, or offers practice in body weight support gait training to improve walking.

There is nothing in the law that specifically states that modalities cannot be used in school-based practice. Legal decisions support a district's choice of intervention as long as the district is able to verify that the student is making progress toward IEP goals with the intervention provided. Below are some questions to help guide therapists in deciding whether to use a modality as an intervention for a student at school.

- Modalities often focus on an impairment area rather than a student's functional level, so what is the functional outcome (IEP goal) that the modality supports?

- Is there a different therapy intervention that could help the student reach the same functional outcome?

- Is there a safe place to use the equipment?

- Who will supply and fund the equipment (school, student's insurance)?

- Where will the equipment be stored?

- How will the equipment be maintained?

- Who will maintain and inspect the equipment?

- In the context of evidence-based practice, is there evidence to support the use of the modality?

- What data will be collected to demonstrate the student's response to the modality?

- Does the student show progress in terms of functional outcomes and IEP goals?

Motor Control, Motor Learning, and Motor Development

PTs help students solve movement problems. In order to do this, PTs must have an understanding of the scientific theories and research in the areas of motor control, motor learning, and motor development. The following is adapted with permission from Patricia C. Montgomery, Ph.D., PT, FAPTA from her presentation, *Motor Control, Motor Learning, and Motor Development: Implication for Effective Treatment in Pediatrics.* (October 2003)

Motor Control

Motor control refers to the control of posture and movement as part of a dynamic system. System models consider multiple variables that influence motor behavior. Instead of a fixed set of equilibrium reflexes, contemporary system models consider postural responses as flexible, functional motor skills that can adapt with training and experience. A child's postural responses are proactive, centrally organized, and based on prior experience and intention. The implication for intervention is to facilitate balance in a variety of tasks and contexts.

Contemporary system models consider postural responses as flexible, functional motor skills that can adapt with training and experience.

In contemporary system theories, functional motor behaviors are critical within the context of a meaningful environment. The PT analyzes the student's postural and movement skills in the context of the school environment. This approach aligns with IDEA 2004 and the emphasis on the student's functional performance. The PT sees how the student is able to control posture and balance in the classroom, hallways, lunchroom, playground, gymnasium, and school grounds. The PT may work with the student on developing ankle strategies, hip strategies, stepping, or grasping to maintain posture and balance, and on integrating and practicing these motor behaviors in routines within the school setting.

Motor Learning

Motor learning is the acquisition of a motor behavior or skill achieved by periods of practice and experience. Motor learning is in contrast to motor performance. Motor performance is a skill learned during a practice session, which does not result in long-lasting change. Motor learning is a set of processes for acquiring capability for producing skilled action that lasts and that is part of everyday function. Motor learning is a direct result of practice and is relatively permanent.

Variables that assist motor learning include:

1. Comprehension of the task through verbal instruction, demonstration, modeling by other students or practice

2. Motivation through activity that is meaningful or functional

3. Practice, practice, practice

4. Attention and effort

5. Specific goal setting with the student's involvement

6. Knowledge of results

7. Random practice rather than concentrating on a single task, especially with children

8. Learning the activity in environment where it naturally occurs

9. Practicing the task in multiple settings to avoid difficulties in generalizing or transferring skills to a new setting

10. Cooperation and competition

11. Mental practice such as social stories before trying the task or skill

12. Feedback from movement errors

Motor learning lends itself to integrated therapy where motor skills are practiced in the environment in which the task naturally occurs. As such, integrated therapy offers practice opportunities and supports motivation and attention.

Motor Development

Motor development refers to changes in motor behavior during a person's life span. In the context of the enablement (ICF) model, motor development is considered part of health, fitness, and life-long leisure skills.

School-based PTs require knowledge of the development of gross motor functional movement from early childhood through young adulthood. New, documented research indicates that there is no single best developmental sequence. Development is simultaneous, not strictly sequential. Therapeutic interventions include age-appropriate activities based on the child's chronological age and interest. Instead of the therapist providing *hands-on treatment*, the therapist guides the movement or task and then allows the student to learn movement through trial and error, making the student an active participant in therapy. Preschoolers develop movement patterns or motor programs as part of play. Practice rolling, crawling, creeping, and climbing can be embedded in a gross motor obstacle course in the preschool class or daycare. School-age children refine gross and fine motor skills through practice and in response to challenges in physical education, sports, music, recess, and the classroom. The student may practice moving with crutches up and down classroom aisles, hallways, and ramps. For high school students, transition plans may include part of community participation, recreation, and leisure. For example, the PT may work with a student on developing the motor skills needed to open and close the car door and to get in and out of the car so the student can begin drivers education.

Instead of the therapist providing hands-on treatment, the therapist guides the movement or task and then allows the student to learn movement through trial and error, making the student an active participant in therapy.

Evidence-Based Practice and Critical Inquiry

IDEA 2004 requires that special education and related services must be based on "peer-reviewed research to the extent practicable." "Scientifically-based research means research that involves the application of rigorous, systematic, and objective procedures to obtain reliable and valid knowledge relevant to education activities and programs." (20 USC sec. 7801(37)) This corresponds to evidence-based practice in physical therapy. Evidence-based practice in physical therapy evolved from the move to evidence-based medicine. Evidence-based medicine is defined as "the integration of best research evidence with clinical expertise and patient values."

Evidence-Based Practice

The five steps of evidence-based practice for a PT are:

1. Formulate the clinical question.

2. Obtain the evidence with searches.

3. Evaluate the evidence for clinical validity.

4. Combine evidence with clinical judgment.

5. Evaluate the fidelity of implementation. Fidelity refers to providing the intervention in a way that compares favorably with the original design of the evidence-based practice. (American Physical Therapy Association 2007, 1-3; Ottenbacher and Cusick 1990)

Levels of evidence come from the hierarchies developed in medicine to "rate the strength of the research designs being used to generate the evidence." D. L. Sackett, et al. (2000) are usually cited as the source of this approach, although similar hierarchies appear across the healthcare literature. Research design levels from strongest to weakest are

I   Strong evidence from at least one systematic review of multiple, well-designed, randomized, controlled trials

II   Strong evidence from at least one properly designed, randomized, controlled trial of appropriate size

III Evidence from well-designed trials without randomization, single group, pre-post, cohort, time series, or match case-controlled studies

IV   Evidence from well-designed non-experimental studies from more than one center or research group

V   Opinions of respected authorities, based on clinical evidence, descriptive studies, or reports of expert committees

Levels of evidence come from the hierarchies developed in medicine to rate the strength of the research designs being used to generate the evidence.

Besides research design, the other factors to appraise are sample size, internal validity, and external validity. Sample size is rated A (sample size greater or equal to 20) or B (less than 20). Internal validity is rated 1 (high), 2 (moderate), or 3 (low). External validity is rated a (high), b (moderate), or c (low). Research with the strongest evidence is IA1a. (Cope 2005)

How is the busy school-based PT able to find the time to apply an evidence-based approach to day-to-day practice? Some school-based therapists address this challenge by forming therapy groups to research a practice issue. Therapists in the Waukesha School District collectively develop a clinical question and then individually search for evidence in one article to answer this question. Each therapist reviews one article, rates the level of evidence, and reports the findings at the next therapists' meeting. In this way, therapists learn from several articles and discuss the application of this evidence to practice.

Concordia University of Wisconsin and a private practice group, Dominiczak Therapy Associates LLC, both based in the Milwaukee area, partnered to explore evidence-based practice. Dominiczak Therapy Associates contracts with school districts to provide school-based therapy services. The Dominiczak Therapy Associates' therapists developed clinical questions. Concordia University DPT (Doctor of Physical Therapy) students from the Tools for Evidence-Based Practice class (taught by Kathryn Zalewski, PT, Ph.D.) researched and reviewed the literature for articles addressing the clinical questions and then rated the level of evidence in the articles. Concordia and Dominiczak expanded this collaboration by inviting school-based PTs, OTs, and directors of special education to attend a half-day presentation on Evidence in School-Based Therapy. The DPT students shared their evidence-based practice findings on therapeutic interventions used by school-based therapists. This collaboration is an innovative way for therapists to learn about evidence guiding and informing practice and for the therapists to earn continuing education credits.

Journals and databases provide access to articles and summaries of evidence. The Occupational Therapy and Physical Therapy pages on the Wisconsin DPI website provide a link to online databases for finding abstracts and citations for individual articles and systematic reviews. Professional organizations provide access to evidence. Members of the American Physical Therapy Association (APTA) can access *Hooked on Evidence* and other resources from the APTA website as well as receive professional journals which contain recent research on effective interventions.

Continuing education courses are another means for therapists to keep current on evidence-based practice. To assure that course content is evidence-based and not just the presenter's opinion, the therapist may request that the instructor provide supporting evidence for course content.

Choosing Interventions

School-based PTs use activity-focused motor interventions for children in preschool and school-based settings. Activity-focused interventions involve structured practice and repetition of functional actions and are directed toward the learning of motor tasks that will increase the student's participation in daily

Besides research design, the other factors to appraise are sample size, internal validity, and external validity.

routines. Activity-focused motor interventions are integrated in everyday classroom and school activities. (Rapport 2009) The PT chooses interventions based upon

- IDEA, which emphasizes functional performance.

- peer-reviewed research and evidence-based practice.

- contemporary research on motor control, motor learning, and motor development.

- preferred practice patterns (*Guide to Physical Therapist Practice*).

- enablement models, which emphasize function, participation, and community integration.

When parents disagree with the choice of intervention, court rulings have supported districts' choices of methodology or intervention. If a district offers a student an appropriate educational program, it can choose the methodology. Under IDEA, districts do not have to document a particular methodology or intervention on a student's IEP. Instead, the IEP team addresses the student's goals, not a particular intervention. This gives the therapist more flexibility in trying new strategies to meet the student's needs and changing status. However, districts must be able to verify that the student is making progress toward IEP goals with the intervention provided. Data collection and progress monitoring are ways to document progress. With peer-reviewed research in IDEA 2004, PTs may corroborate the selection of a particular intervention based upon evidence in research. Parents may pursue private therapy or community-based services for a particular intervention, in addition to the therapy the school district provides.

Progress Reports and Re-examination

According to the APTA's *Guide to Physical Therapist Practice,* PTs routinely perform *re-examinations* of a student's progress to modify or redirect interventions. This may include the student's response to intervention, communication with staff or others, progression, precautions, and plans for the next session. Re-examination corresponds to IDEA's requirement that the IEP team informs parents about their child's progress on IEP goals. PTs contribute to the IEP team progress report to parents.

Discontinuation

As noted in chapter 3, dismissal from physical therapy occurs when the student no longer requires the therapy to benefit from special education. "The results of a recent nationwide survey of school-based PTs found that the most important factor in determining service termination was whether the student met functional goals. This is accepted professional practice and aligns with discontinuation of

Activity-focused motor interventions are integrated in everyday classroom and school activities.

other IEP services. This study also found that the influence of the parents/caregiver was usually the most difficult factor in discontinuing physical therapy. Therapists need to continually collaborate with parents to foster understanding and trust and help prepare parents for termination of services." (Effgen 2000, 12:121-26.) The *Guide to Physical Therapist Practice* states that PTs provide a summation of the outcome of physical therapy services at the point of discontinuation of therapy. In school-based practice this would include noting the student's progress, current functional status, and goal achievement (IEP goal that the therapist supported). Documentation requirements that are part of special education and physical therapy practice follow.

Post-high School Transition

One of the stated purposes of IDEA is to prepare children with disabilities for further education, employment, and independent living. *Transition service* means a coordinated set of activities for a child with a disability that

- is designed to be within a results-oriented process.

- is focused on improving the academic and functional achievement of the child with a disability to facilitate the child's movement from school to post- school activities, including post-secondary education, vocational education, integrated employment (including supported employment), continuing and adult education, adult services, independent living, or community participation.

- is based on the individual child's needs, taking into account the child's strengths, preferences, and interests.

- includes instruction, related services, community experiences, the development of employment, and other post-school adult living objectives, and, when appropriate, acquisition of daily living skills and functional vocational evaluation.

Recognizing that starting the transition planning early is important, Wisconsin law requires the IEP team to develop post-secondary goals for a student at age 14 rather than waiting until age 16 as required by IDEA. The district invites the student to the IEP meeting as the student's input is vital. Transition planning is an opportunity for the student to begin thinking about or deciding career choices, training needs, employment possibilities, and housing options post-high school. When the student is unable to attend, the IEP team considers the student's preferences and interests. An IEP team member meets with the student to discuss the student's plans for post-high school and brings the information to the IEP meeting. Parental involvement in transition planning is essential as an opportunity for parents to consider what life will be like for their child post-high school, and to have a voice in decisions.

Therapists need to continually collaborate with parents to foster understanding and trust and help prepare parents for termination of services.

Assessment tools include criterion-referenced assessments, student interest surveys, structured ecological assessments, and observations in natural contexts. These assessments help the entire team evaluate the student in the areas of training, education, employment, and independent living skills. Examples of criterion-referenced instruments are the Enderle-Severson Transition Rating Scale-Third Edition (ESTR III), which is designed for learners with moderate to severe disabilities, and the Enderle-Severson Transition Rating Scale-Form J-Revised, which is designed for learners with mild disabilities. Both evaluate student performance in the areas of employment, recreation and leisure, home living, post-secondary education, social/vocational behavior, and community participation. Teachers, parents, therapists, and the student complete the assessment, which identifies the student's strengths, the areas requiring assistance, and the ongoing supports the student will require to participate in post-high school environments.

Based upon the specific transition issues from the assessment, the IEP team collaboratively determines outcomes and writes these as measurable goals in the IEP. Goals address high school completion; productive activity including community employment, supported employment, or post-secondary education; community leisure involvement including friendship and community participation; and community living. The team looks for opportunities that offer direct experience in real life for work, social interaction, and a place to live. Opportunities may be at school, home, work, or the community. The team considers accountability in terms of student outcomes through periodic review of the student's actual performance. (Spencer 2006)

The team looks for opportunities that offer direct experience in real life for work, social interaction, and a place to live.

PTs are uniquely qualified to be a part of the IEP team as PTs understand

- Function and performance.

- Activity demands and contexts.

- Effects of disability.

- Self-sufficiency and self-determination.

- Accommodation, modification, and adaptation.

Figure 21 on the following page shows effective intervention approaches for youth in transition.

Figure 21 Effective Intervention for Youth in Transition

Type of Physical Therapy Intervention	Examples of Interventions in Transition
Teaching skills, habits, behaviors	Provide motor learning opportunities for mobility in the community and using public transportation
Compensation/adaptation • Changing task: objects, methods • Changing environment: social, physical • Training others to support	Use biomechanics for positioning and assistive technology to access the environment. Recommend modifications such as grab bars in restrooms, ramps for access Collaborate with community-based agency staff and offer training
Preventing disability	Educate students about prevention of secondary impairments
Promoting health	Develop lifelong fitness activities for the student

Documentation

School-based PTs must meet documentation requirements for special education and for physical therapy practice. Special education laws require that the PT

- develop IEP goals with the team.

- contribute to progress reports on IEP goals.

- provide written information that can be used in developing or revising the IEP when physical therapy will be discussed at an IEP meeting but the PT is excused from attending.

- develop a physical therapy treatment plan.

- provide a written policy and procedure for written and oral communication for general supervision of a physical therapist assistant (PTA).

The Practice Act requires the PT to create and maintain a patient record for every patient that the PT examines or treats. The content of the patient record is not defined. Direction is given in the *Guide to Physical Therapist Practice* which states the *Guidelines for Physical Therapy Documentation* include

- initial examination and evaluation.

- intervention or service provided.

- status, progress, or regression.

- reexamination and reevaluation.

- discontinuation of service or episode of care.

Even though IDEA 2004 no longer requires a summary of findings, the PT may write an evaluation report. The local district may develop a form for this purpose. Other helpful recordkeeping includes regular, ongoing documentation of each child's physical therapy intervention and the child's response. Standard documentation for school physical therapy also includes

- attendance records that document the amount and frequency of service that therapist provides to the child.

- progress notes on intervention plans and data collection on IEP goals.

- notes on contacts with parents, physicians, teachers and vendors.

- summation of care (discharge summary).

Records help the PT focus on educationally relevant intervention as well as provide helpful background and historical treatment information when a child transfers from one therapist to another. Records form a basis for the PT to assess the quality of the service and determine typical amounts of therapy needed to accomplish similar outcomes with other children. Medical assistance and other medical insurance providers may require PTs to keep other specific records to obtain third-party payment for physical therapy.

Communication

The school PT communicates with students, families, school staff, and outside agencies. PTs motivate students by communicating clearly at age-appropriate levels and with cultural sensitivity. PTs contribute to good parent and school relationships by providing parents with updates on their child's progress. A telephone call, e-mail message, or note home in the student's backpack is a quick and efficient way to keep parents informed about how their child is doing. The PT helps build collaborative teams by avoiding jargon and by using active listening skills when working with school staff. Effective communication with administrators is clear, concise, and supported with data and evidence.

A telephone call, e-mail message, or note home in the student's backpack are quick and efficient ways to keep parents informed about how their child is doing.

The PT also bridges communication between the educational and medical communities. The school PT can help health care providers understand the school district's services and legal responsibility to provide physical therapy. When physicians and other health care providers furnish medical information to the school, the PT summarizes and interprets the information related to physical therapy for students, families, caregivers, and school staff. The school PT also can share with medical providers' information about the child's function at school, need for adaptive equipment, and any changes in the child's physical status that may require further diagnostic intervention.

Fitness and Health

PTs design prevention, fitness, and wellness activities. Therapeutic exercise is part of fitness and wellness programs. PTs may design exercise to promote overall health or prevent complications due to inactivity or overuse of muscles and joints. School therapists design and modify fitness and health as part of universally designed programs for all students, as selective options for some students, or as a targeted, individualized program for a student with a disability. APTA's FUNfitness is a screening kit to assess children's flexibility, strength, and balance and is designed for children and youth with and without disabilities. FUNfitness was initially developed for the Special Olympics *Healthy Athletes* program. (APTA 2001)

IDEA 2004 includes universal design as a means to maximize access to general education curriculum for all students. *Universal design* involves designing and delivering products and services that are usable by all people with the widest possible range of functional capabilities. An example of a program with universal design that the school PT provides is the backpack program to prevent back pain and stress for all students. When the PT collaborates with the physical education instructor to develop curriculum that provides fitness activities for students with varying levels of strength, stamina, and endurance is also an example of universal design. This curriculum offers options so students can select activities that match or challenge their fitness level. The PT might participate on a district-wide committee for playground design or redesign and choice of equipment to allow for accessibility by many students.

In Wisconsin public schools, physical education must be made available to all children, including children with disabilities. Physical education is required for children with disabilities when the school provides it to their peers or when the IEP team determines the student needs physical education. The IEP team determines whether the student receives regular, adapted, or specially designed physical education. The PT can measure the child's flexibility of arms and legs, functional strength of abdominal and leg muscles, and balance. The PT may collaborate with the physical education instructor to adapt the gym environment, equipment, or curriculum so the student is able to participate in wellness and fitness activities in regular or specially designed physical education. The PT and physical education teacher can design an individualized program tailored to provide aerobic conditioning to meet the child's fitness needs.

PTs design prevention, fitness, and wellness activities.

Privacy

It is accepted practice in a clinical setting for a patient to partially disrobe during evaluation or intervention. This allows the PT to observe joint alignment, palpate for muscular contraction, and assess movement. The school PT may need to ask a child to remove some clothing to perform an accurate evaluation, examination, or intervention. The removal of a child's clothing during a physical therapy evaluation or intervention session may raise concerns in the school setting. Some children, parents, and administrators have questioned the practice, and some therapists are concerned about accusations of sexual abuse. To avoid these misunderstandings, the district can implement these policies:

- During the orientation process, the special education director discusses with the PT the accepted practices for disrobing children and providing hands-on therapy in the school setting. PTs who previously worked in a hospital or clinical setting especially need to discuss these practices.

- At school, the child dresses in regular school clothes for most physical therapy.

- The child brings gym clothes, shorts, and T-shirt for the therapy sessions.

- The district provides a setting that allows for appropriate privacy, especially for evaluation sessions.

- The therapist explains to the parent and child prior to an evaluation or therapy session that at times partial disrobing of the child may be part of the assessment and hands-on therapy.

- Districts prepare a written policy to share with staff and parents, and ask for signed, parental permission prior to a hands-on physical therapy evaluation and intervention.

- The district invites parents to observe the physical therapy evaluation and intervention.

- Another school staff member is present during the evaluation or examination.

Ethics

APTA established a code of ethics for PTs and standards of ethical conduct for PTAs. APTA offers accompanying guides for professional conduct for PTs and PTAs. PTs and PTAs are responsible for maintaining and promoting an ethical practice. Responsibilities to the consumer, the profession, the law, the public, and themselves underlie the principles that make up these documents. Chapter PT 9, Wis. Admin Code reinforces the importance of ethical conduct by requiring four hours of continuing education in ethics and jurisprudence for biennial license renewal.

It is a professional expectation that PTs and PTAs who work in the school will promote the welfare of children and strive for excellence in practice.

It is a professional expectation that PTs and PTAs who work in the school setting will adhere to the principles guiding the profession in a manner that will promote the welfare of children and strive for excellence in practice. Appendix D contains the *APTA Code of Ethics for the Physical Therapist* and the *Standards of Ethical Conduct for the Physical Therapist Assistant.*

Cultural Competency

Therapists need to be cognizant of cultural influences on the development of a child's motor skills and the values parents place on disability and therapeutic interventions. Therapists "…must recognize the influences of culture in the development of gross motor skills. Data generated by such instruments may need to be interpreted with caution when assessing a child of different cultural backgrounds and should always be used in conjunction with other evaluative measures to determine levels of gross motor development." (Cohen, et al. 1999, 197) In this study, "the sample of children of African American background consistently achieved more gross motor skills at an earlier age than the established normal values (norms). The children of Hispanic background scored closer to the normative data in most skill categories." (Cohen, et al. 1999, 191) Therapists need to exercise caution when interpreting standardized measures of a student's motor skills and consider the student's cultural background.

In a recent study of "Values Anglo-American and Mexican-American Mothers Hold for Their Children with Physical Disabilities," Elizabeth Mae Williamson concludes, "therapists should consciously seek to build strong professional relationships and establish open, honest communication between themselves and all caregivers. An understanding of what values are important to individual families and recognition of perceived and true difficulties confronted by individual families may reduce the covert influence of societal distinction on the habilitative process." (Williamson 2002, 21)

References

Allen, D. 2007. "Proposing 6 Dimensions within the Construct of Movement in the Movement Continuum Theory." *Physical Therapy* 87(7):888-98.

American Physical Therapy Association. 1999. *Guide to Physical Therapist Practice.* Alexandria, VA: American Physical Therapy Association.

___. 2001. "FUNfitness: A Screening Kit to Assess Children's Flexibility, Strength, and Balance." Alexandria, VA: American Physical Therapy Association.

___. 2007. "Evidence-based Practice in Pediatric Physical Therapy." Section on Pediatrics FACT SHEET. http://www.pediatricapta.org/consumer-patient-information/pdfs/Evidence-based%20Practice%20Fact%20Sheet.pdf (Accessed April 5, 2010 members only).

Birmingham, G., et al. 2006. *Pennsylvania Physical Therapy Association Guidelines for the Practice of Physical Therapy in Educational Settings.* Pennsylvania Physical Therapy Association Pediatric Special Interest Group.

Cecere, S. 7/25/07. "Re: assessment tools." ped-pt@listserv.temple.edu Section on Pediatrics. American Physical Therapy Association.

Cohen, E., K. Boettcher, T. Maher, A. Phillips, L. Terrel, K. Nixon-Cave, and K. Shepard. 1999. "Evaluation of the Peabody Developmental Gross Motor Scales for Young Children of African American and Hispanic Ethnic Backgrounds," *Pediatric Physical Therapy* 11(4):197.

Cope, S. "Using Systematic Reviews to Inform Practice." Presented at the Statewide School Therapy Conference, Wisconsin Dells, WI, October 28, 2005.

Coster, W., T. Deeney, J. Haltiwanger, and S. Haley. 1998. *School Function Assessment.* San Antonio, TX: Pearson.

Effgen, S. 2000. "Factors Affecting the Termination of Physical Therapy Services for Children in School Settings." *Pediatric Physical Therapy* 12(3):121-26.

Enderle, J. and S. Severson. 2003. Enderle-Severson Transition Rating Scale, 3rd Ed. Moorhead, MN: ESTR Publications.

Montgomery, P. 2003. "Motor Control, Motor Learning, Motor Development: Implications for Effective Treatment in Pediatrics." Presentation at Statewide School Therapy Conference. Wisconsin Dells, WI.

Ottenbacher, K.J. and A. Cusick. 1990. "Goal Attainment Scaling as a Method of Clinical Service Evaluation." *American Journal of Occupational Therapy* 44: 519-525.

Rapport, M. 2009. "Activity-Focused Motor Interventions with Children in Preschool and School-Based Settings." APTA Learning Center. PT Baltimore 2009 Revisited.

Sackett, D.L, W.S. Richardson, W.M.C. Rosenberg, and R.B. Haynes. 2000. Evidence-based Medicine: How to Practice and Teach EBM. 2nd Edition. London: Churchill-Livingstone.

Spencer, K. "Related Services and Transition." Presented at the Statewide School Therapy Conference, Wisconsin Dells, WI, October 27, 2006.

Williamson, E. 2002. "Values Anglo-American and Mexican-American Mothers Hold for Their Children with Disabilities." *Pediatric Physical Therapy* 14(1):16-21.

World Health Organization. 2002. "Beginner's Guide: Towards a Common Language for Functioning, Disability and Health ICF," http://www3.who.int/icf/icftemplate.cfm?myurl=introduction.html%20&mytitle=Introduction (page discontinued, see below).

World Health Organization. "International Classification of Functioning, Disability and Health, ICF." http://www.who.int/classifications/icf/en/ (accessed March 9, 2010).

Other Resources

American Physical Therapy Association. 2001. *Topics in Physical Therapy: Pediatrics*, Alexandria, VA: American Physical Therapy Association.

___. 2008. *Topics in Physical Therapy: Pediatrics, Vol.2.* Alexandria, VA: American Physical Therapy Association.

Asbjornslett, M. and H. Hemmingsson. 2008. "Participation at School as Experienced by Teenagers with Physical Disabilities." *Scandinavian Journal of Occupational Therapy* 15:153-61.

Darragh, A., M. Campo, and D. Olson. (in press). "Safe patient handling: A qualitative study of occupational and physical therapists." *Work: A Journal of Prevention, Assessment, and Rehabilitation.*

Darragh, A., W. Huddleston, and P. King. 2009. "Work-Related Musculoskeletal Disorders in OTs and PTs." *American Journal of Occupational Therapy.*

Effgen, S. 2005. *Meeting the Physical Therapy Needs of Children.* Philadelphia, PA: F.A. Davis Company.

Effgen, S., L. Chiarello, and S. Milbourne. 2007. "Updated Competencies for Physical Therapists Working in Schools." *Pediatric Physical Therapy* 19(4):266-74.

Hanft, B. and P. Place. 1996. *The Consulting Therapist.* San Antonio, Texas: Therapy Skill Builders, a division of the Psychological Corporation.

Hanft, B., D. Rush, and M. Shelden. 2004. *Coaching Families and Colleagues in Early Childhood.* Baltimore: Paul H. Brookes.

"Intervention for Youth Who Are in Transition from School to Adult Life." 2006. Developed by the Practice Committee of the Section of Pediatrics, APTA, with special thanks to expert contributors A. Doty and L. Sylvester. Section on Pediatrics Fact Sheet. Alexandria, VA: American Physical Therapy Association.

Jette, A. 2005. "The Changing Language of Disablement." *Physical Therapy* 85(2):118-19.

McEwen, I. and M. Rapport. 2009. *Providing Physical Therapy Services Under Parts B & C of the Individuals With Disabilities Education Act (IDEA).* Alexandria, VA: Section on Pediatrics, American Physical Therapy Association.

Rehabilitation Engineering & Assistive Technology Society of North America (RESNA) Position. "The Application of Power Wheelchairs for Pediatric Users," http://www.rstce.pitt.edu/RSTCE_Resources/Resna_position_on_Peds_wheelchair_Users.pdf (accessed March 16, 2010).

The Special Educator. "Don't 'Lock' Your District into Specific Methodology." *LRP Publications* 23(18):6.

Supervision of Assistants and Other Personnel

6

Occupational therapists (OTs) and physical therapists (PTs) follow specific requirements in state law when supervising other personnel hired by school districts to assist in the provision of occupational therapy and physical therapy. Supervised personnel may include licensed occupational therapy assistants (OTAs), licensed physical therapist assistants (PTAs), licensed special education aides, and students performing fieldwork in fulfillment of university and technical college programs. Supervision involves guidance and oversight related to the delivery of occupational and physical therapy services for which the respective therapists are responsible. Unlike collaborative intervention, which is described in more detail in chapter 7, supervision requires personnel to deliver occupational therapy or physical therapy in schools following the direction and instruction of the respective therapist who supervises the therapy itself. This occurs after the collaborative process of the IEP or other team has determined the therapy needed.

OTAs and PTAs are educationally prepared to assist the respective therapists in providing effective and cost-efficient services.

Occupational Therapy Assistants and Physical Therapist Assistants

In response to a critical shortage of OTs and PTs to provide services to students, DPI promulgated administrative rules, effective July 1, 1993, to license OTAs and PTAs to work in public schools. OTAs and PTAs are educationally prepared to assist the respective therapists in providing effective and cost-efficient services. Both are graduates of two-year technical colleges and are licensed by the Department of Regulation and Licensing (DRL) as well as by DPI.

Occupational Therapy Assistants

An occupational therapy assistant (OTA) provides occupational therapy under the close or general supervision of an OT. The OT in collaboration with the OTA determines the level of supervision. This determination is made on the basis of the training and experience of the OTA, the familiarity of the OTA with school-based practice, and the nature of the therapy required by specific children. No one other than an OT can legally delegate occupational therapy treatment to an OTA.

An OTA may collect data and assist with evaluations, but it is the responsibility of the OT to conduct, interpret, and report on evaluations. Essentially, the OTA shares the OT's caseload. The OTA provides therapy according to a written treatment plan that the OT alone or in collaboration with the OTA is required to develop. Following the establishment of service competence, the OTA may provide any facet of treatment that the OT delegates. Service competence is defined later in this chapter. The responsibility for the outcomes of the therapy provided by the OTA remains with the OT.

Supervision requirements for the school-based OTA are found in Chapter PI 11, Wis. Admin Code and correspond with Chapter OT 4, Wis. Admin Code rules. The details of supervision and caseload are provided in Figure 22 on pages 131 and 132. The supervising OT writes both a policy and procedures that the OT will follow when supervising the OTA, including the procedure for written and oral communication. The written procedures include each child's name, status and plan, and these may be incorporated into the child's treatment plan. Levels of supervision are either close or general. Under close supervision, the school OT must have daily, direct contact on the premises with the school OTA. The OT co-signs evaluation and intervention documents prepared by the OTA. Close supervision is required for all school system services provided by an entry-level OT. Entry-level means the person has no demonstrated experience in a new position or in school system practice. The duration of close supervision is determined by the supervising OT, based on service competence of the OTA. Under general supervision, the OT must reevaluate the occupational therapy of each child assigned to the OTA at least once a month or every tenth treatment day, whichever is sooner. The OTA does not have to be present. The OT and the OTA must meet face-to-face, with or without the child present, every fourteen calendar days to discuss progress, problems, or other issues relating to the provision of school occupational therapy. These requirements assure that the OT remains familiar with every child on the caseload in order to monitor progress, adjust treatment to the child's needs, and contribute to IEP planning.

The OTA may not represent an OT on an IEP team. The OTA may attend the IEP meeting, but only with the supervising OT present. It is highly likely that the IEP team will ask the assistant to participate in program development, which the assistant may not do without the supervising therapist. Many schools are reluctant to use both the therapist's time and the assistant's time for the same IEP meeting because of cost. The OTA often sees the students for therapy while the OT attends IEP meetings, to avoid cancelling therapy sessions that the district has an obligation to provide.

Licensure Requirements

OTAs are licensed by the Occupational Therapists Affiliated Credentialing Board (OTACB), which is part of the DRL. OTAs must successfully complete the academic requirements and supervised internship of an accredited educational program in occupational therapy. All OTAs must complete two written examinations, and an oral examination may be required. The written examinations are the *National Board or Certification in Occupational Therapy Examination for Occupational Therapy Assistants* and an open book examination on the Wisconsin Statutes and Administrative Code. An OTA must renew a DRL license every two years. The OTA must complete 24 hours of continuing education for license renewal during this period. To work in schools, the OTA must have a current DRL license, complete the application process for a license from the DPI, and obtain the DPI license. Chapter 2, Figure 4 describes DRL licensure requirements.

The OTA provides therapy according to a written treatment plan that the OT alone or in collaboration with the OTA is required to develop.

Physical Therapist Assistants

The PTA provides physical therapy under the direction and supervision of a PT. The PTA provides selected components of physical therapy intervention, obtains data related to that intervention, makes modifications in interventions as directed by the PT or to ensure the student's safety, and interacts with staff and others. The PT delegates those portions of a child's physical therapy which are consistent with the PTA's education, training, experience, and skill level. The PT considers the criticality, acuity, stability, and complexity of the child's condition or needs. The PT also considers the predictability of the response to intervention. After taking all of these factors into account, the PT determines the safe and appropriate level of supervision of the PTA. Interventions that are exclusively performed by a PT and cannot be delegated include but are not limited to spinal and peripheral joint mobilization/manipulation, which are components of manual therapy, and sharp selective debridement, which is a component of wound management. These interventions are typically not part of school-based practice.

Supervision requirements for the school-based PTA are found in Chapter PI 11, Wis. Admin Code and correspond to Chapter PT 5, Wis. Admin. Code. The details of supervision and caseload are provided in Figure 22 on pages 131 and 132. Requirements include a written policy that describes the procedure for written and oral communication. The policy and procedures also describe the specific supervisory activities that the PT undertakes for the PTA. Levels of supervision are either close or general. Close supervision requires that the PT has daily, direct contact on the premises with the PTA. General supervision means that the PT has direct face-to-face contact with the PTA at least every 14 calendar days. This could be at the school with the PTA and student present or this could be offsite with just the PT and PTA present. The PT provides onsite reevaluation of each child's therapy a minimum of one time per calendar month or every tenth day of service, whichever is sooner and adjusts the therapy plan as appropriate.

Responsibilities of the PT include examination, evaluation, and reevaluation of the child, participation in the development of the child's IEP, and development of the intervention plan. The PTA may assist with data collection but cannot administer tests.

The PTA documents interventions performed, data collected, student progress, equipment provided, and communication with others. However, the PTA may not interpret this information. The PTA signs the documentation. The documentation may be a narrative form, checklist, flow sheet, or graph, determined by the PT. The PT authenticates all documentation. One such method has the PT review the documentation of the PTA monthly and then sign and date each review. These documentation guidelines come from the *Guide to Physical Therapist Practice,* Appendix 7-3 (APTA 1999) and are not found in Chapter PI 11, Wis. Admin. Code or Chapter PT, Wis. Admin. Code. This is best practice, not administrative rule.

The PTA may interact with the child, family, or community providers and participate with the PT in training teachers and other educational staff. The PTA may assist in the design and fabrication of equipment or adaptations for specific

The PTA provides selected components of physical therapy intervention, obtains data related to that intervention, and makes modifications in interventions as directed by the PT.

children as well as participate in departmental planning and management. As such, the assistant takes part in developing internal policies and procedures, helps with budget development, and participates in discussions regarding schedules and assignment of children. The PTA may be assigned a number of responsibilities unrelated to children, including the maintenance of an inventory and budget records, and ordering equipment and supplies.

The PTA may not represent a PT on an IEP team. The PTA may attend the IEP meeting, but only with the supervising PT present. It is highly likely that the IEP team will ask the assistant to participate in program development, which the assistant may not do without the supervising therapist. Many schools are reluctant to use both the therapist's time and the assistant's time for the same IEP meeting because of cost. The PTA often sees the students for therapy while the PT attends IEP meetings, to avoid cancelling therapy sessions that the district has an obligation to provide.

Licensure Requirements
PTAs are licensed by the Physical Therapy Examining Board (PTEB), which is part of the DRL. PTAs must graduate from a program accredited by an agency approved by PTEB. All PTAs must complete a written examination and an oral examination may be required. The written examination is the National Physical Therapist Assistant Examination. Passing scores are those recommended by the Federation of State Boards of Physical Therapy. A PTA license from the DRL must be renewed every two years. The PTA must complete 20 hours of continuing education for license renewal, with 4 hours in ethics and jurisprudence. To work in schools, the PTA must have a current DRL license, complete the application process for a license from DPI, and obtain the DPI license. Figure 4 in chapter 2 summarizes DRL licensure requirements.

School OTAs and school PTAs must work under the close or general supervision of the respective school therapist.

Summary of Supervision
School OTAs and school PTAs must work under the close or general supervision of the respective school therapist. Only a PT or a PTA may provide physical therapy. Only a PT may supervise the physical therapy provided by a PTA. Similarly, only an OT or an OTA may provide occupational therapy. Only an OT may supervise the occupational therapy provided by an OTA. When a full-time OT or PT works with a licensed assistant, the therapist's caseload may increase from a maximum of 30 to a maximum of 45 children.

Figure 22 Supervision of Assistants

	OTA Supervision	PTA Supervision
Delegation	OT determines which occupational therapy services to delegate to the OTA based on service competence. Service competence means the determination made by various methods that two people performing the same or equivalent procedures will obtain the same or equivalent results. OT delegates only those portions of a child's occupational therapy which are consistent with the OTA's education, training, and experience.	PT determines which physical therapy services to delegate to the PTA. PT delegates to the PTA only those portions of a child's physical therapy which are consistent with the PTA's education, training, and experience. PT considers the criticality, acuity, stability and complexity of the student's condition/needs. PT determines the safe and appropriate level of supervision.
Close supervision	Required for all school system services provided by an entry-level OTA. *Entry-level* means OTA has no demonstrated experience in a specific position: a new graduate, a person new to the position, or a person in a new setting with no previous experience in that area of practice. OT has daily, direct contact on the premises with OTA. No standard exists for duration of close supervision other than *service competence*.	PT has daily, direct contact on premises with the PTA.
General supervision	OT has direct, face-to-face contact with the OTA at least once every 14 calendar days. Between direct contacts, OT is available by telecommunication. OT has face-to-face, onsite reevaluation of each child's occupational therapy a minimum of one time per calendar month or every tenth day of occupational therapy, whichever is sooner.	PT has direct, face-to-face contact with the PTA at least once every 14 calendar days. Between direct contacts, the PT is available by telecommunication for direction and supervision. PT provides onsite reevaluation of each child's therapy a minimum of one time per calendar month or every tenth day of service, whichever is sooner and adjusts the therapy plan as appropriate.

	OTA Supervision	**PTA Supervision**
Written policy	Includes procedure for written and oral communication. Specific description of the supervisory activities undertaken for each OTA. Includes client name, status and plan for each client discussed.	Includes procedure for written and oral communication. Specific descriptions of the supervisory activities undertaken for each PTA.
Documentation	When close supervision is required, OT inspects actual implementation of treatment plan periodically. OT cosigns evaluation contributions and intervention documents that the OTA develops.	PTA documents and signs each therapy session in narrative form or uses a checklist, flow sheet, or graph. Elements of documentation include the student's status, progress, or regression as well as interventions and equipment provided. PT authenticates documentation by co-signing.
Caseload	45 based on the OT's full-time equivalency (FTE). A full-time OT is employed for a full day, five days a week. A 1.0 FTE OT may supervise no more than 2.0 FTE OTA positions and no more than 3 OTAs in total. For instance, if the OTA is .50 FTE, a supervisory OT must be in the district at least .25 FTE.	45 based on the PT's full-time equivalency (FTE). A full-time PT is employed for a full day, five days a week. A 1.0 FTE PT may supervise no more than 2.0 FTE PTA positions and no more than 3 PTAs in total. For instance, if the PTA is .50 FTE, a supervisory PT must be in the district at least .25 FTE.
Responsibilities of Supervising Therapist	Overall delivery and outcome of occupational therapy services. Safety and effectiveness of the services provided. Evaluation and reevaluation of the child and interpretation of data. Participation in development of the child's IEP. Development of the treatment plan.	Examination, evaluation, and reevaluation of the child. Participation in the development of the child's IEP. Development of the treatment plan.
Responsibilities of Assistant	OTA may collaborate with OT in evaluation and program planning. OTA may not represent OT on an IEP team.	PTA may assist with data collection, but cannot administer tests. PTA may modify an intervention as directed by the PT or to ensure the child's safety. PTA may not represent a PT on an IEP team.

Service Competence

A positive, collaborative, and student-centered relationship between therapists and assistants depends on a shared view of their respective roles. A therapist new to working with an assistant is sometimes concerned about delegating interventions, as the therapist is responsible for the outcomes of the service delegated to the assistant. Service competence provides a way to ensure a unified approach to the provision of occupational or physical therapy services. Service competence means the determination made by various methods that two people performing the same or equivalent procedures will obtain the same or equivalent results. (Chapter OT 1, Wis. Admin Code) Both the therapist and assistant benefit from a mutually designed system of establishing service competence. Each brings a unique set of skills from which the other can learn. The systematic description of assessment and intervention procedures, and the observation of each other's performance can improve the skills of both.

Service competence provides a way to ensure a unified approach to the provision of therapy services.

The methods chosen for establishing service competence vary. The therapist and assistant begin by determining which interventions are likely to be delegated and are of a high priority. Next, they outline a process for determining service competence. For example, an assistant learning an unfamiliar intervention may

- read about the intervention in an article or book, or online.

- observe the therapist providing the intervention.

- watch recorded sessions of children receiving the intervention.

- co-treat with the therapist so that each can discuss questions.

- provide intervention while the therapist observes.

Preparing a checklist of principles of techniques together ensures that both therapist and assistant address necessary aspects of the intervention. Specific problem areas are noted and revisited until both are satisfied that the chosen approach has established service competence. Three consecutive occasions in which competence has been demonstrated is one possible standard to establish initial competence. After that, the therapist and assistant may periodically co-treat for review or for new approaches. Appendix F includes sample position descriptions for OTs, OTAs, PTs and PTAs.

Non-Licensed Personnel and Occupational Therapy

Non-licensed personnel, in the context of the provision of occupational therapy, refers to individuals who are not licensed as OTs or OTAs by the Department of Regulation and Licensing. This includes teachers who are licensed to provide general or special education, but are not licensed to provide occupational therapy, and paraprofessional teaching assistants. Under Wisconsin law, only a licensed OT or licensed OTA can provide or claim to provide occupational therapy. (s.448.961, Wis. Stats.) The clearest application of this is in the amount and frequency of occupational therapy on a child's IEP, which only an OT or an OTA may deliver. Teachers and paraprofessional teaching assistants make accommodations and prepare a child for activities that take place on a daily basis in the classroom or other school environments. When an OT designs the accommodations and preparation that will be implemented by others, the OT must ensure that they are specific tasks that are within the capacity of teachers and paraprofessional teaching assistants. Neither an OT nor an OTA is permitted to delegate maintenance or restorative tasks that require the judgment, decision-making or skill of an OT. (OT 4.05, Wis. Admin Code) Figure 23 on the following page summarizes the supervision requirements for non-licensed personnel.

Non-Licensed Personnel and Physical Therapy

In the context of the provision of physical therapy, *non-licensed personnel* are individuals who are not licensed as PTs or PTAs. In both cases, this includes teachers and paraprofessional teaching assistants. Teachers and paraprofessional teaching assistants are DPI-licensed personnel under Chapter PI 34, Wis. Admin Code, but they are not licensed by the DRL to provide physical therapy. School personnel sometimes ask if teachers and paraprofessional teaching assistants can assist students with school activities and routines that incorporate motor learning. A student's motor skills are not solely the domain of physical therapy, as these skills fall within the larger context of school functions that all children perform. As described in the School Function Assessment (Coster et al. 1998), students travel throughout the school environment, maintain and change positions, move up and down stairs, manipulate objects while moving, and participate in recreational activities. PTs collaborate with teachers and paraprofessionals to provide accommodations, adaptations, or strategies that help the student participate in classroom routines and school activities. "Other team members whom a PT teaches do not provide physical therapy services. Rather, they carry out educational activities that the PT recommends to help a child learn motor skill, function more effectively in the classroom, and so forth. This should not become a concern when goals are discipline free and reflect a student's overall educational program. Classroom assistants, for example, do not work on *physical therapy goals*." (McEwen 2009, 111–12)

A student's IEP goal may be to transfer from the wheelchair to the toilet with assistance of one person. Initially, the PT works with the student on interventions and strategies that allow the student to move from the wheelchair to the toilet. Intervention may start with strengthening and balance activities and progress to instruction in using adaptive equipment such as a raised toilet seat or grab bars. When the student learns how to perform the transfer safely, the PT teaches the paraprofessional and teacher how to assist a student with moving from wheelchair to toilet. During the training, the PT provides direct, on-premise supervision. When the student has learned the safe transfer skill, it is a school function in bathroom hygiene. It is no longer a physical therapy intervention and the PT discontinues providing direct service toward this goal. The paraprofessional helps the student with the transfer under the supervision of the teacher

Non-licensed personnel refers to individuals who are not licensed as OTs, OTAs, PTs or PTAs. This includes teachers and paraprofessional teaching assistants.

as part of school routines. At that time, the IEP may include adult assistance for all toilet transfers as a supplementary aid and service.

The IEP team determines when physical therapy is required for a student to achieve an IEP goal. The PT then determines the physical therapy intervention, whether the intervention can be delegated to a PTA, and when an activity or task is part of classroom or school routines. The IEP team documents the PT's time to train and collaborate with classroom teachers and paraprofessionals in the student's IEP under Program Modifications or Supports for School Personnel.

The details of delegation and supervision of non-licensed personnel in the provision of occupational therapy and physical therapy as specified in the Wisconsin Administrative Code are provided in Figure 23 on this page.

Figure 23 Supervision of Non-Licensed Personnel

	Non-Licensed Personnel Occupational Therapy	**Non-Licensed Personnel Physical Therapy**
Supervision	Must be under direct supervision of OT or OTA at all times. Must be in immediate area and in audible and visual range of supervisor for maintenance and restorative tasks.	Must be under the direct, on-premises supervision of the PT at all times.
Delegation or Instruction	Performs only non-skilled, specific tasks. May not receive delegation of any direct client care which requires an OT's judgment or decision-making.	Performs tasks which do not require a PT's clinical decision making or PTA's clinical problem solving.
Collaboration	Collaborates with OT, client, family, caregiver or other involved individuals or professionals when OT evaluates and provides intervention. Receives education from OT along with client, family, caregiver or others in carrying out appropriate non-skilled strategies.	Collaborates with PT and other educators when PT supports the student's IEP goal with adaptations, accommodations, and strategies that allow a student to participate in classroom activities or routines.
Designation	May not designate self as occupational therapist, occupational therapy assistant, OT, OTR, OTA, or COTA or claim to render occupational therapy.	May not designate self as physical therapist or claim to render physical therapy.

Clinical Affiliations and Training Opportunities

A crucial way to maintain the supply of school OTs and school PTs is for public schools to offer clinical affiliations and fieldwork experiences for student OTs, PTs, OTAs and PTAs under the supervision of school therapy staff. Without on-the-job training opportunities in school districts, future school therapists and assistants may have experience only in medically based settings. School districts sometimes find that upon graduating and receiving a license, the therapy student they trained is a welcome candidate to fill a vacant therapy position.

Student Occupational Therapists and Occupational Therapy Assistants

School-based OTs may accept student OTs and student OTAs for fieldwork experiences. School-based occupational therapy fieldwork educators may participate in meetings of Wiscouncil (Wisconsin Council on Occupational Therapy Education), a consortium of the five OT educational programs and the five OTA educational programs in Wisconsin. Regional Fieldwork Educators Certificate Workshops designed by the American Occupational Therapy Association (AOTA) are hosted periodically by Wiscouncil members. AOTA has numerous resources available to fieldwork educators and others at www.aota.org. School-based fieldwork experiences allow students to learn by working with an experienced therapist, practice newly acquired skills, and become familiar with school-based therapy as a possible career choice. The responsibilities of the fieldwork educator include planning the student's experience, orienting the student to school-based practice, supervising the student's experience, and evaluating the student's performance. In exchange for training opportunities, students enrich staff by sharing their enthusiasm and bringing knowledge of current evidence, research, and therapy interventions.

Licensure Requirements

Student OTs and student OTAs do not need a license to participate in fieldwork experiences. S.448.962 (1)(b), Wis. Stats. establishes that a license is not required for "any person pursuing a supervised course of study, including internship, leading to a degree or certificate in occupational therapy under an accredited or approved educational program, if the person is designated by a title which clearly indicates his or her status as a student or trainee." A similar statement in s.448.962(2)(b), Wis. Stats. applies to student OTAs.

Supervision of the Student Occupational Therapist and Student Occupational Therapy Assistant

Occupational therapy fieldwork experiences in public schools may be at Level 1 or Level 2. The purpose of Level 1 fieldwork is to introduce students to the fieldwork experience and develop a basic comfort level and understanding of the needs of children with disabilities in school. Level 1 fieldwork is not intended to develop independent performance of the student OT or OTA, but to enrich class work through directed observation and participation in selected aspects of the occupational therapy process. The student OT and OTA should be supervised in all aspects of the fieldwork experience with full knowledge of and responsibility by the supervisor.

Level 2 fieldwork prepares the student OT and OTA to assume the responsibilities of an entry-level OT or OTA. The supervising OT should provide supervision daily as an essential part of the fieldwork program. It should be flexible in accordance with the interests, needs and abilities of the OT or OTA student. Supervision should begin with direct supervision and gradually decrease to less direct supervision as the student demonstrates competence with respect to the setting and children's conditions and needs. Supervision includes direct observation of the interaction between the therapy student and the child, role modeling, meetings with the student, review of student paperwork, consultation and communication regarding the learning experience.

New Graduates

School districts may hire new graduates but must be aware of licensure and supervision requirements. An OT or OTA *may not practice* in any setting in Wisconsin without a temporary or permanent license from the DRL in his or her possession. An OT or OTA who is a graduate of an approved school and is scheduled to take the national certification examination for OT or OTA, or has taken the national certification examination and is awaiting results, may apply to the OTACB in the DRL for a temporary license. Practice during the period of the temporary license must be in consultation with an OT who endorses the activities of the person holding the temporary license on at least a monthly basis. An OT or OTA with a temporary license may practice at no more than two separate employment locations. A temporary license expires on the date the applicant is notified that he or she has failed the national certification examination, the date the board grants or denies an applicant permanent licensure, or the first day of the next regularly scheduled national certification examination for permanent licensure if the applicant is required to take, but failed to apply for, the examination. The OT or OTA with a temporary DRL license may apply for a one-year license from the DPI to work in schools. DPI changes the one year license to a five-year license when the OT or OTA receives the regular DRL license.

School districts may hire new graduates but must be aware of licensure and supervision requirements.

Student Physical Therapists and
Student Physical Therapist Assistants

School-based PTs may accept student PTs and student PTAs for clinical affiliations or training sessions. The Wisconsin Clinical Education Consortium (WCEC) offers basic clinical instructor workshops and credentialing workshops that school-based PTs may attend. School-based clinical affiliations allow students to learn by working with an experienced therapist, practice newly acquired skills, and become familiar with school-based therapy as a possible career choice. The responsibilities of the clinical PT instructor include planning the student's experience, orienting the student to school-based practice, supervising the student's experience, and evaluating the student's performance. In exchange for training opportunities, students enrich staff by sharing their enthusiasm and bringing knowledge of current evidence, research, and therapy interventions.

Licensure Requirements

Student PTs and student PTAs do not need a license to participate in clinical affiliations or training sessions. The Physical Therapy Practice Act at s.448.52(1m)(c), Wis. Stats. states that a license is not required for "a physical therapy student assisting a physical therapist in the practice of physical therapy or a physical therapist assistant student assisting a physical therapist in performing physical therapy procedures and related tasks, if the assistance is within the scope of the student's education or training."

Supervision of the Student Physical Therapist and Student Physical Therapist Assistant

There are two requirements of the school-based PT when supervising student PTs. First, the PT must be present physically and immediately available for direction and supervision during the student's interaction with the child. Second, the PT must interact with the child within a 24-hour period each time the student PT provides services to the child. The PT could be in the same room, in the near vicinity, or on a different floor of the school building as long as the PT is immediately available for the student if needed. Being available by telecommunication does not meet the requirement.

These same two requirements apply to the supervision of the student PTA whether the PT is supervising the student PTA alone or in conjunction with a school-based PTA. Again, the PT must interact with the child within a 24-hour period each time the student PTA provides services to the child and the PT must be present physically and immediately available for direction and supervision. When the school-based PTA in conjunction with the PT supervises the student PTA, the PT must be on the premises. If the PT is not on the premises, the student PTA can observe the PTA but cannot provide any intervention. The PT must co-sign or authenticate all student PTA documentation.

New Graduates

School districts may hire new graduates but need to be aware of licensure and supervision requirements. A PT or PTA who is a graduate of an approved physical therapy or PTA program may apply to the Physical Therapist Examining Board (PTEB) in the DRL for a temporary license. The duration of a temporary license is three months or until the holder receives examination results, whichever is shorter. A PT or PTA may renew a temporary license for a period of three months, and may renew it a second time for a period of three months for reasons of hardship. So, PTs and PTAs may practice under a temporary license for not more than a total of nine months. The PT or PTA with a temporary DRL license may apply for a one-year license from the DPI to work in schools. DPI changes the one-year license to a five-year license when the PT or PTA receives the regular DRL license. If the PT or PTA fails the licensing examination, the PT or PTA no longer can work in schools as a provider of physical therapy.

The school-based, licensed PT must provide direct, immediate, and on-premises supervision of a PT or a PTA with a one-year DPI license and temporary DRL license, including authenticating documentation.

The school-based, licensed PT must provide direct, immediate, and on-premises supervision of a PT or a PTA with a one-year DPI license and temporary DRL license.

References

American Physical Therapy Association. 1999. *Guide to Physical Therapist Practice, Second Edition.* Alexandria, VA: American Physical Therapy Association. Chapter 1, Appendix 2, 4, 5, 7.

Coster, W., T. Deeney, J. Haltiwanger, and S. Haley. 1998. *School Function Assessment.* . San Antonio, TX: Pearson.

McEwen, Irene. 2009. *Providing Physical Therapy Services Under Parts B & C of the IDEA.* Second Edition. Alexandria, VA: Section on Pediatrics, American Physical Therapy Association.

Wisconsin Department of Regulation and Licensing. "Occupational Therapy Assistant." http://drl.wi.gov/profession.asp?profid=29&locid=0 (accessed August 18, 2010).

___. "Physical Therapist Assistant." http://drl.wi.gov/profession.asp?profid=38&locid=0 (accessed August 18, 2010).

Other Resources

American Physical Therapy Association. 2000. "Procedural Interventions Exclusively Performed By Physical Therapists." American Physical Therapy Association Position Paper (HOD P06-00-30-36).

___. 2000. "Provision of Physical Therapy Interventions and Related Tasks." American Physical Therapy Association Position Paper (HOD-P06-00-17-28).

___. 2005. "Direction and Supervision of the Physical Therapist Assistant." American Physical Therapy Association Position Paper (HOD P06-05-18-26).

___. 2007. *A Normative Model of Physical Therapist Assistant Professional Education: Version 2007.* Alexandra, AV: American Physical Therapy Association.

Bezner, J. "Supervision and Best Practice." December 2001. *PT Magazine* 9(12): 22–24. Alexandria, VA: American Physical Therapy Association.

Black, T. and K. Eberhardt. 2005. *The Occupational Therapy Assistant.* Bethesda, MD: AOTA Press.

Rainforth, B. and J. York-Barr. 1997. *Collaborative Teams for Students with Severe Disabilities.* 2nd ed. Baltimore: Paul H. Brookes.

Schuh, M. 2002. "Student Supervision: Legal, Ethical and Reimbursement Considerations." *Wisconsin Clinical Education Consortium Clinical Education Newsletter 1–2.*

Steffes, L. and B. Winiecki. 2007. "Wisconsin Physical Therapy Practice Act and Rules: Regarding Physical Therapy Assistants." *PT Connections*. WPTA Newsletter 37(1): 9–10.

"Student Physical Therapist Provision of Services." 2000. American Physical Therapy Association Position Paper (HOD P06-00-18-30).

"Supervision of Student Physical Therapist Assistants." 2000. American Physical Therapy Association Position Paper (HOD P06-00-19-31).

Tomczyk, K. November 2000. "Practice." *PT Connections*. WPTA Newsletter 30(6): 5–7, 14.

Watts, N. T. 1971. "Task Analysis and Division of Responsibility in Physical Therapy." *Physical Therapy* 51: 23–35.

Wisconsin Department of Public Instruction. "Occupational Therapy." http://dpi.wi.gov/sped/occ_ther.html (accessed August 18, 2010).

___. "Physical Therapy." http://dpi.wi.gov/sped/phy_ther.html (accessed August 18, 2010).

___. "Frequently Asked Questions about School Occupational Therapy and School Physical Therapy." 2008. http://dpi.wi.gov/sped/pdf/otpt-faq-overview.pdf (accessed August 18, 2010).i

Collaborative Service Provision

7

Collaborative service provision strengthens the skills and effectiveness of team members as they invest their time in learning about each other's roles and analyzing how they can integrate multiple and varied intervention approaches. This will increase the magnitude and effectiveness of intervention. (Rainforth and York-Barr 1997) Because the educational process is a dynamic system that involves the child and others who interact with the child, collaborative intervention can create outcomes that are more useful for the child and valued by all who are involved with the child.

Collaboration in School for Children with Disabilities

The IEP team decides what services a child with a disability will receive. Hanft and Place (1996) recommend that service and role decisions begin by identifying

- desired student outcomes, reflected in IEP goals.

- strategies that facilitate the outcomes.

- the necessary expertise to implement the strategies.

- the best method of service delivery.

An IEP team often determines that a special education teacher or teaching team can implement strategies on a daily basis. When the teachers and student need the expertise of an occupational therapist (OT) or physical therapist (PT) to help with designing or implementing strategies, the IEP team may suggest collaborative consultation. In collaborative consultation, the child's teachers and therapists work together to identify daily needs and develop and implement strategies. This differs from expert consultation, in which the specialist independently evaluates needs, develops interventions, and provides one-on-one intervention or makes recommendations to staff. Current research supports collaborative consultation over expert consultation. Whether or not an OT or PT works directly with a child, collaborative consultation in which the teacher and therapist act as co-equals should be part of the child's therapy.

Current research supports collaborative consultation over expert consultation.

Integrated Therapy

Collaborative consultation lends itself to implementing educationally relevant, functional activities so that the child practices newly acquired skills during naturally occurring routines and environments. Known as integrated therapy, it is coordinated within the routines of the special education or regular education classroom. Integrated therapy allows the PT to incorporate opportunities for the student to practice newly acquired movement in daily school activities and routines. With these embedded interventions, the student is afforded multiple opportunities to practice motor skills in purposeful ways. Integrated therapy allows the OT to establish or restore a child's performance skills or patterns when and where they are needed, and to help the child develop strategies for daily task or activity performance. With integrated therapy the child

- practices and learns skills in the place he will use them.

- practices skills in naturally occurring routines.

- has increased practice opportunities.

- has increased opportunities for social relationships.

- engages in regular classroom routines.

- does not miss out on classroom activities.

The student is afforded multiple opportunities to practice skills in purposeful ways.

In addition to these advantages for the child, the intervention team benefits from integrated therapy in the following ways.

- Therapists can see whether or not the strategies are working in the classroom.

- Teachers and therapists focus on skills that are immediately useful for the child.

- Teachers can build their capacities and skills based on what works for children.

- Therapists and teachers can work together to address problems as they arise. (McWilliam 2010)

Location, the focus of the above lists, is only one of several characteristics of integrated therapy. Other factors include the presence of peers, the frequency of activities, transitions between activities, the functionality of skills, and opportunities for collaborative consultation.

Some strategies that the teacher and therapist design may not require the therapist's expertise, so the teacher or other staff person may provide them. This model of service delivery is indirect, because the therapist's knowledge and skills benefit the child without direct interaction. When the therapist's expertise is required to safely and effectively provide an intervention, the therapist provides the intervention. This is a clinical decision that the PT makes about physical therapy interventions, and the OT makes about occupational therapy interventions. Interventions of this type may require an understanding of human anatomy, physiology, biomechanics or neurology that a teacher or paraprofessional would not be expected to have. This model of service delivery is direct. Individual direct service occurs when the therapist works with a child, one-on-

one. The PTA and OTA, under the supervision of the respective therapist, may also provide direct service. Many parents will assume that occupational therapy and physical therapy are always direct and one-on-one. Although not required by law, writing on the IEP whether service is direct or indirect clarifies the service for parents. Direct service may or may not be integrated into the child's typical routines and environments.

Based on the experience of school-based therapists and action research projects in the state, direct service by the therapist within the classroom is easiest to do in preschool and early elementary grades. At higher grade levels, physical education class may be an appropriate context for direct service by the therapist. Physical therapy or occupational therapy may help the child benefit from integrated practice of movement components such as strength, flexibility, speed, adaptability, endurance, eye-hand coordination, or motor planning in the gym, pool, or weight room as part of the physical education curriculum. Community activities, independent living skills or work experiences that are part of a youth's transition services may include direct services by a therapist to build physical capacity, adapt to new environments or learn new skills. Through collaborative consultation, the therapist and teachers can develop strategies for students to practice new learning in a meaningful way as part of the transition activities and real-life experiences.

At higher grade levels, physical education class may be an appropriate context for direct service by the therapist.

Sometimes the IEP team may decide that direct intervention by the therapist in a separate setting is the best way for the child to achieve desired outcomes. Selection of the setting depends on many factors, including the

- need for the child to have privacy.

- distractibility of the child.

- activity or skill involved.

- child's level of learning in a particular skill.

- child's learning style.

- potential for disruption of other students.

Studies have found that school-based PTs and OTs recommended a combination of integrated and isolated services, supporting the value of both approaches. (Kaminker 2006; Rainforth and York-Barr 1997) The varieties of models and teacher involvement in Figure 24 on the following page serve as a tool for therapists to identify the models of service delivery they typically use and consider if integrating services to a greater degree would be appropriate for a child.

Figure 24 Continuum of Service Delivery Models

Model	Location	Therapy Focus	Peers	Teacher's Role
Individual Pull-Out	Anywhere apart from the regular class	Directly on child functioning	Not present	Provide information before therapy and receive information after therapy
Small Group Pull-Out	Anywhere apart from the regular class	Directly on functioning by children with special needs	One to six peers present	Provide and receive information before & after therapy, decide schedule with therapist & which peers will participate
One-on-one in Classroom	Classroom, often apart from other children	Directly on child functioning	Present but not involved in therapy	Conduct activities, play with other children, keep children from disrupting therapy; rarely, watch therapy session, provide and receive information after therapy
Group Activity in Classroom	Classroom; small or large group	On all children in group and on peer interactions, emphasis on meeting special needs of children	All or some children in group have special needs	When small group, conduct activities and play with other children; if possible, watch or participate in therapist's group. When large group, watch or participate in group activity and participate in planning large and possibly small group activity
Individual During Routines	Classroom, wherever focal child is	Directly but not exclusively on the focal child	Usually present	Plan and conduct activity including focal child, observe therapist's interactions with child, provide information before therapy, exchange information with therapist after routine
Collaborative Consultation	In or out of classroom	Teacher, as related to the needs of the child; can vary from expert to collegial model	Present if occurring in class; not present if occurring out of class	Exchange information and expertise with therapist, help plan future therapy sessions, give and receive feedback, foster partnership with therapist

From McWilliam, R. A. 1995. "Integration of therapy and consultative special education: A continuum in early intervention." *Infants and Young Children*, 7(4), 29-38. Reprinted with permission.

The varieties of models and teacher involvement serves as a tool for therapists to identify the models of service delivery they typically use.

Assistive Technology

Another way that school OTs and school PTs collaborate with other school personnel may be through providing an assistive technology service. The IEP team considers whether or not the student requires assistive technology devices and services. The district ensures that assistive technology devices or assistive technology services are made available to a child with a disability if required as part of special education, related services, or supplementary aids and services. The term *assistive technology service* refers to any service that directly assists a child with a disability in the selection, acquisition, or use of an assistive technology device. (34 CFR s. 300.6) Assistive technology service includes

- evaluating the needs of a child with a disability, including a functional evaluation of the child in his or her customary environment.

- purchasing, leasing, or otherwise providing for the acquisition of assistive technology devices for children with disabilities.

- selecting, designing, fitting, customizing, adapting, applying, maintaining, repairing, or replacing assistive technology devices.

- coordinating and using other therapies, interventions, or services with assistive technology devices, such as those associated with existing education and rehabilitation plans and programs.

- training or technical assistance for a child with a disability, or, if appropriate, that child's family.

- training or technical assistance for professionals (including individuals providing education and rehabilitation services), employers, or other individuals who provide services to, employ, or are otherwise substantially involved in the major life functions of that child.

Therapists often participate in evaluating a child's need for assistive technology.

OTs often participate in evaluating a child's need for assistive technology. An OT who performs any part of such an assessment specific to an individual child must do so through the IEP team process unless the child is currently receiving occupational therapy. The OT will use the results of the evaluation as the basis for the selection and modification of devices, as well as training of the child and others in the use of the devices. Occupational therapy roles that do not involve assessment or recommendations for a specific child, such as assessing the building, providing general information about devices and services, or facilitating group decision-making do not require an IEP team evaluation or reevaluation process.

PTs have a role in determining the need for and the selection of many types of assistive devices. These professionals also train others in the use of assistive technology devices. A PT who performs any part of such an assessment specific to an individual child must do so through the IEP team process unless the child is currently receiving physical therapy.

An erroneous assumption is that assistive technology refers only to computers or augmentative communication systems. Specialized devices for feeding, dressing, toileting, enhancing mobility, transferring, maintaining and changing position in the classroom, cooking, holding books, and writing are examples of the many assistive technology devices that children with disabilities may need in school. The online database known as AbleData (National Institute on Disability and Rehabilitation Research, U.S. Dept. of Education) provides a reference for over 36,000 product listings in 20 categories.

Equipment Use by Other School Staff

Recent complaints investigated by DPI regarding a positioning chair, stander, and weighted blanket highlight the need for the IEP team to consider the safety of individual students and issues of restraint when including assistive technology devices on a student's IEP. In order to ensure that assistive technology, adaptive equipment or other therapeutic equipment is not considered a mechanical restraint, a health care provider (PT, OT, or physician) recommends or prescribes the device for a specific child and the child's IEP team makes the decision for its use. Adaptive equipment, belts, and fasteners are for postural support and stability and are not to be used for behavior management. Instead, a functional behavioral assessment (FBA) and a positive behavioral intervention plan (BIP) are ways school staff address a student's behavioral needs. For detailed information, see DPI Directives for the Use of Seclusion and Physical Restraint in Special Education Programs at http://dpi.wi.gov/sped/sbseclusion.html.

Assistive Technology Policies and Procedures

While the IEP team focuses on the assistive technology needs of the individual student, the district needs a written policy and procedures for the overall general use of equipment. Appendix E includes a sample district policy. (Kutschera 2009) Some districts develop guidelines for use of specific equipment such as *Guidelines for the Use of Weighted Blankets and Vests* in Appendix E. District policy

- includes documentation of equipment procedures for individual students.

- addresses the ongoing training plan for teachers and staff members.

- identifies the population to be served, activities that will be supported, and settings in which equipment will be used.

- outlines the administrative approval process.

- identifies storage areas.

- establishes a maintenance schedule.

- ensures equipment use in accordance with manufacturer's specifications.

- requires a copy of the manufacturer's specifications attached to the equipment so it is not lost or misplaced. (Darragh and Hussey 2008)

Adaptive equipment, belts, and fasteners are for postural support and stability and are not to be used for behavior management.

A picture of the student in the equipment verifies its use according to manufacturer's specifications and serves as a reference for staff. Sample forms for trial equipment, equipment usage, monthly equipment check, and logging use and response are in Appendix E.

Safe Handling and Lifting Technology

In addition to the safety of students when they are lifted or repositioned, districts consider the safety of staff when moving and positioning students. Neither the DPI nor the Wisconsin Department of Workforce Development has rules, policies, or guidelines on weight restrictions for lifting students or for determining when a lifting device is necessary. New research on worker injuries provides data for instructing staff on how to assist students with disabilities with transfers, gait, and repositioning. In industry, lifting a load of greater than 50 pounds is considered a risk for injury. Due to the different characteristics of lifting and moving people, lifting a person who weighs more than 35 pounds is considered a risk factor for injury. Ergonomic variables to consider when lifting students are the size of the student, level of assistance required, purpose, frequency, location, and the student's own unpredictable movement while being lifted.

Ergonomic variables are the size of the student, level of assistance required, purpose, frequency, location, and the student's own unpredictable movement while being lifted.

District policies and procedures, staff position descriptions, or union-management agreements may address the amount of weight that staff may lift when moving or transferring students. Collaborative development of a local lifting policy protects staff from injury that occurs from cumulative trauma and overexertion. Purposes of safe handling methods are to

- achieve goals with less risk and less physical effort of all staff.

- increase availability of teachers to focus on education rather than physical support.

- increase availability of the therapist to focus on therapeutic interventions.

The trend in many health care facilities is for staff to use a mechanical lifting device. Mechanical lifts can be electric or hydraulic, have sling supports, and have a mobile base or track system. Some equipment that is available for positioning or mobility includes gait trainers, body weight support devices, standers, and sit-to-stand devices. Friction reducing devices are available to help with transfers. The Occupational Safety and Health Administration (OSHA 2009) provides algorithms that assist in decision-making regarding lifting, positioning, and transferring individuals.

Safe Transportation

A student's specific transportation plan may be part of the student's IEP or in a separate individualized health plan (IHP). An IHP is more readily revised to meet changing circumstances and needs. The therapist collaborates with other school personnel, the student's family and the student in the development of a safe transportation plan by recommending equipment, providing personnel training, and advising on procedures for picking up and dropping off the student. If the student can be transferred safely from the wheelchair and positioned on the bus seat or requires a car seat, the therapist recommends specific modifications for bus seating or may instruct staff in positioning, transfer techniques, and use of equipment. A trial run of the equipment and route helps make sure that the plan provides for safe transportation. It also allows students and staff to become familiar with the procedures and ask questions or share concerns. The American Academy of Pediatrics (2010) provides a resource, *Car Safety Seats: A Guide for Families,* which offers information on height and weight limits for car seats and travel vests. The American Academy of Pediatrics (2008) also provides a policy as part of *School Bus Transportation of Children with Special Health Care Needs.*

When the student will be transported in a wheelchair on a bus or van, the wheelchair must be secured and the occupant wears a seatbelt. Wheelchairs and strollers are not designed as motor vehicle seats and an unsecured wheelchair is a danger to the occupant and other students. The IEP team considers wheelchair tie down and occupant restraint system (WTORS). The WTORS secures the wheelchair and provides the student with a properly designed and tested seatbelt system. Figure 25 on the next page provides guidelines for safe transportation of students in wheelchairs.

The Wisconsin Department of Transportation administrative rules specify transportation of school children. Power lifts or ramps, wheelchair fasteners, and seats and restraints are found at Chapter Trans 300.76-78, Wis. Admin Code.

Emergency Evacuation

A student's emergency evacuation plan provides for the student's safe exit from a building. The therapist participates in development of the plan, the selection of mechanical devices, positioning strategies, and handling techniques. Lifting and carrying the student may seem expedient but the team should consider possible injury to the student or staff, as well as the student's self-esteem, dignity, and independence. An alternative for the team to discuss is the use of a special evacuation chair. The Fire Department may designate a rescue area that is identified with an emergency sign. In an emergency, the student proceeds or is moved to the designated area or room with a staff person to await rescue.

The team also considers safe evacuation of the student from a school bus or van in case an emergency occurs during transportation. The evacuation plan includes safe handling and movement of the student, identifies any additional equipment needed, and provides for staff training.

Emergency evacuation of students with disabilities falls under emergency nursing services. The Wisconsin Administrative Code requires each school district to provide emergency nursing services under a written policy adopted and implemented by the school board. Emergency evacuation procedures may be found in the local school district policy. Like a student transportation plan, an emergency evacuation plan is part of a student's IEP or separate individualized health plan (IHP). The district invites local emergency personnel from the fire department, police, and EMS to be part of the planning process. (s.121.02(1) (g) Wis. Stats., and PI 8.01(g),Wis. Admin Code)

Like a student transportation plan, an emergency evacuation plan is part of a student's IEP or separate individualized health plan.

Figure 25 Guidelines for Safe Transportation

For safe transportation of students in motor vehicles, The Rehabilitation Engineering Research Center on Wheelchair Transportation Safety recommends the following:

- *Start with the right equipment.* Use a Wheelchair Tiedown and Occupant Restraint System (WTORS) that has been crash tested and labeled as complying with SAE J2249, a voluntary standard developed by safety and rehabilitation experts. The wheelchair should be designed and tested for use as a seat in motor vehicles, often referred to as a WC19 wheelchair. These wheelchairs comply with ANSI/RESNA WC19, a voluntary standard developed by safety and rehabilitation experts. A WC19 wheelchair has four, crash-tested securement points where tiedown straps and hooks can be easily attached. These points are clearly marked with a hook symbol.

- *Secure the wheelchair.* Always position the wheelchair and rider facing forward. Attach the four tiedown straps to the securement points provided on the wheelchair. Tighten the straps to remove all slack. Do not attach tiedowns to adjustable, moving, or removable parts of the wheelchair such as armrests, footrests, and wheels. Remove the wheelchair lap tray and store securely in another area.

- *Protect the student.* To protect the student during a crash or sudden braking, provide the student with a crash-tested lap and shoulder belt or with a child restraint harness. The lap belt should be placed low across the front of the pelvis near the upper thigh, not high over the abdomen. The lap belt should be angled between 45° and 75° to the horizontal. The diagonal shoulder belt should cross the middle of the shoulder and the center of the chest and should connect to the lap belt near the hip of the wheelchair rider. Postural support belts attached to the wheelchair are not strong enough to withstand the force of a crash and are not positioned correctly to restrain the student in a crash.

The therapist recommends specific modifications for bus seating or may instruct staff in positioning, transfer techniques, and use of equipment.

The WC19 website http://www.rercwts.org/RERC_WTS2_KT/RERC_WTS2_KT_Stand/RERC_WTS2_19_Chart.html provides an up-to-date list of wheelchairs and seating systems successfully crash tested with 4-point strap-type securement as of July 27, 2009.

Collaboration in Birth to 3 and Early Childhood

Infants and toddlers may receive occupational therapy or physical therapy in Birth to 3 programs. This program, unique for both its age range and philosophy, is in Part C of the Individuals with Disabilities Education Act. It requires states to provide special education and related services to

> infants and toddlers with disabilities....from birth through age two, who need early intervention services because they (1) are experiencing developmental delays, as measured by appropriate diagnostic instruments and procedures in one or more of the following areas: cognitive development; physical development, including vision and hearing; language and speech development; psychosocial development; or self-help skills, or (2) have a diagnosed physical or mental condition which has a high probability of resulting in a developmental delay. (34 CFR 303)

In Wisconsin, the designated lead agency for the provision of services for children in Birth to 3 programs is the Wisconsin Department of Health Services (DHS). The state agency responsible for special education and related services for children three to twenty-one years old is the Wisconsin Department of Public Instruction (DPI). DHS and DPI have policies and procedures in place for smooth and effective transitions from Birth to 3 to early childhood services. A child's IEP must be in effect no later than the child's third birthday. The district is required to participate in the Transition Planning conference. With the parent's request and consent, the district must invite the Birth to 3 service coordinator to the initial IEP team meeting. Figure 26 on page 152 illustrates the transition timeline of young children from Birth to 3 (Part C) to early childhood special education (Part B).

Wisconsin authorizes a collaborative evaluation process for young children with disabilities. A school district or other local educational agency (LEA) may enter into an agreement with a county Birth to 3 administrative lead agency to allow school employees to participate in evaluations and development of Individualized Family Service Plans for Birth to 3 intervention. The two agencies may also enter into an agreement to allow Birth to 3, Head Start, or tribal school personnel to serve as members of the IEP team and participate in the development of the IEP for early childhood (ages 3 through 5) services (s.115.85 (5) Wis. Stats.) When service providers suspect a child in a Birth to 3 program may need special education in school, they should refer the child for an IEP team evaluation by the age of two years nine months. Coordination between the two programs can begin well before this time.

The same criteria for receiving occupational therapy or physical therapy apply to young children three to five years of age who receive early childhood special education as any other child with an identified educational disability: it is required to assist a child to benefit from special education. It is important, however, to note that occupational therapy and physical therapy provided in a Birth to 3 program are significantly different from school-based occupational therapy and physical therapy. In a Birth to 3 program, occupational therapy and

Occupational therapy and physical therapy provided in a Birth to 3 program are significantly different from school-based occupational therapy and physical therapy.

physical therapy may be *primary* service options, depending on the needs of the child and the family. In the school, occupational therapy and physical therapy are *related* services, provided only when needed to help a child benefit from special education. The criteria are markedly different.

Therapists can take an active role in clarifying for parents how the role of therapy may change as a child makes the transition from the Birth to 3 services into early childhood services. Parents may develop the perception that maintaining a particular amount or type of therapy is the key component in a child's development. It is easy to see how this can happen during the early years of family-centered therapy when, by law and by definition, occupational therapy and physical therapy may be the child's only intervention. Communication among educators, school therapists and Birth to 3 service providers, as well as parents, is essential for a successful transition.

Wisconsin was a part of The National Individualizing Preschool Inclusion Project and continues to promote the continuum of placement options. Placement in natural environments includes three critical components: functional intervention planning, integrated therapy, and embedded intervention. Functional intervention planning is carried out principally through a *routines-based assessment*, featuring an interview of the family and the teaching staff. Integrated therapy consists of specialists using models we have labeled *individualized within routines* and *group activity* to provide special education and related services. *Embedded intervention* involves the use of proven instructional principles, especially incidental teaching, in the context of developmentally appropriate activities. This model is grounded in evidence. As Birth to 3 and early childhood programs incorporate these components into service delivery, the transition from one program to the other may be less disruptive for parents and children.

Collaboration in Private School

Children with disabilities whose parents have enrolled them in private schools have no individual entitlement to receive some or all of the special education and related services they would receive if enrolled in a public school, with the exception of child find, which includes evaluations. After initially evaluating a student and determining the student is eligible for special education, the district where the private school is located should explain to the parents what services are available if the student remains in the private school. If the student remains in the private school and will receive services from the school district, the district develops a *services plan* for the student.

Children with disabilities whose parents have enrolled them in private schools have no individual entitlement to receive some or all of the services they would receive if enrolled in a public school.

Figure 26 Birth to 3 Early Childhood Transition

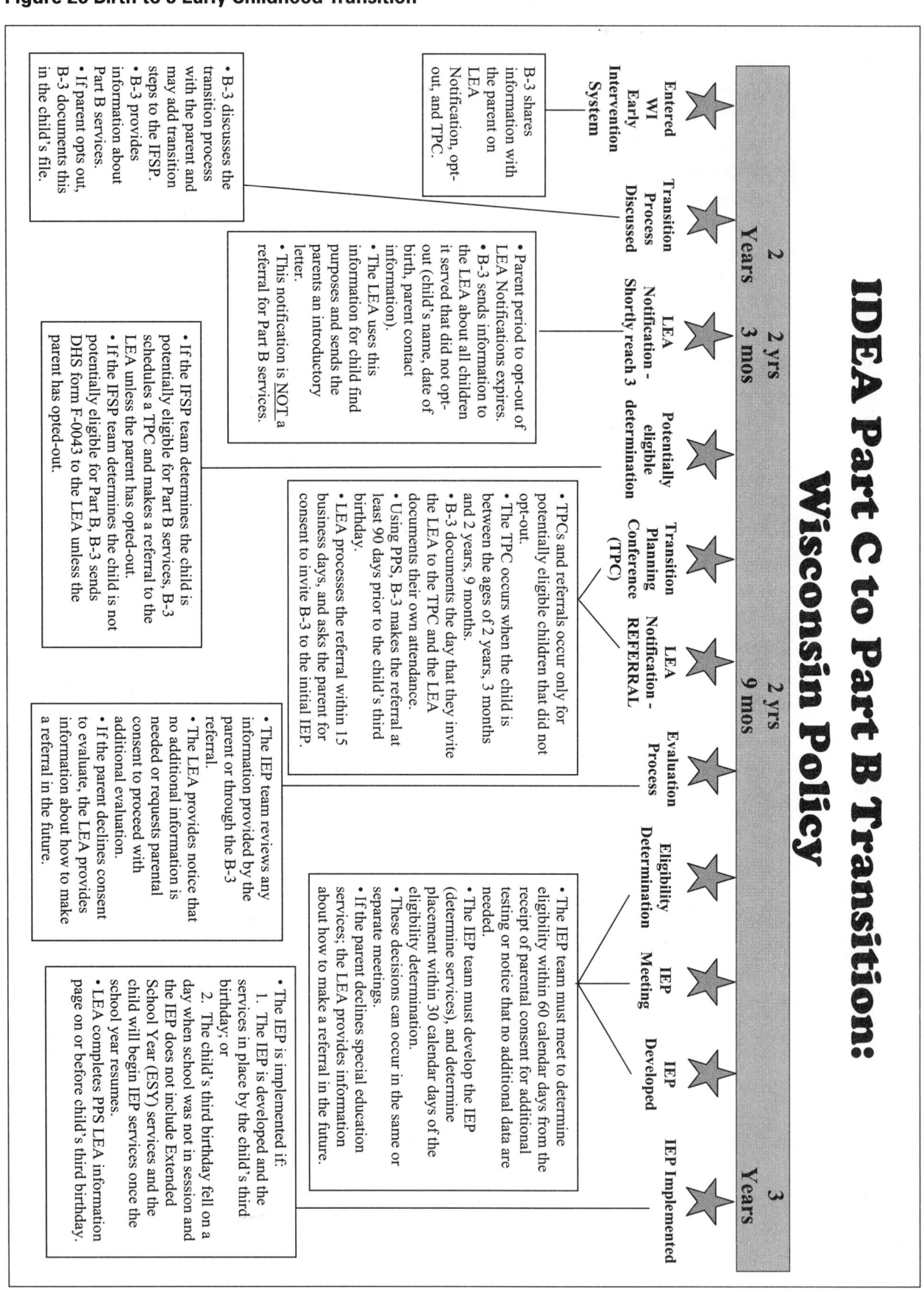

IDEA Part C to Part B Transition:
Wisconsin Policy

The district decides what special education services and related services it will provide to parentally placed private school students with disabilities by consulting in a timely and meaningful way with private school representatives and parents of parentally placed private school students with disabilities. If occupational therapy or physical therapy is a service that a district will provide, the services plan for a student may include occupational therapy or physical therapy. IDEA regulations permit a district to provide for the participation of a private school student in any of the district's special education services. Therefore, the district may provide occupational therapy or physical therapy to the student without providing special education. The therapist may provide services at a private school, including a religious school site.

Home School

Under Wisconsin law, a home-based private educational program (home school) is not a private school. Therefore, the IDEA requirements relating to parentally placed private school students do not apply to children in home school. School districts do not have an obligation to provide special education and related services to children with disabilities enrolled in home school. This includes school-based occupational therapy or physical therapy. However, neither federal nor state law prohibits districts from providing special education and related services to children with disabilities enrolled in home-based private educational programs. School districts are permitted to provide any special education and related services to these children that they deem appropriate. If a public school district chooses to provide these services, the costs are not aided by the DPI under federal or state categorical aids. IDEA requires public school districts to identify and evaluate all children in the district who may have a disability. If the parents of a child in a home-based private educational program suspect that their child may have a disability, they can refer the child for an evaluation at the public school. The district will then perform a publicly funded evaluation of the child and, if found to be a child with a disability, offer the child a placement to meet the child's educational needs. If this child is found to have a disability, the district must offer a placement that would provide the child a free appropriate public education (FAPE). Generally, this placement means the child would be enrolled in a public school.

IDEA requirements relating to parentally placed private school students do not apply to children in home school.

Virtual Collaboration

Telehealth is the use of electronic information and telecommunications technologies to support long-distance clinical health care, patient and professional health-related education, public health and health administration. Technologies used in telehealth typically are: videoconferencing, the Internet, store-and-forward imaging, streaming media, and wired and wireless communications. While new applications are increasingly found for using these technologies, significant barriers remain to making these technologies an integral part of daily health care practice. (Health Resources and Services Administration, 2010)

The term telerehabilitation, on the other hand, means the "clinical application of consultative, prevent[ive], diagnostic and therapeutic therapy via two-way interactive audiovisual linkage." (Scheideman-Miller 2004, 241) It is the real time interaction that separates telerehabilitation from telehealth. Telerehabilitation includes occupational therapy, physical therapy, speech–language pathology, and biomedical engineering services, among others, and covers a broad array of rehabilitation activities, including patient assessment, therapeutic intervention, progress monitoring, education, and training. (Russell 2007)

DPI does not endorse specific service delivery models or practices. Districts are required to provide FAPE in the least restrictive environment (LRE) to all children enrolled in special education in the district. On a case-by-case basis, as part of the individualized education program (IEP) team process, the IEP team determines the special education services (including service delivery) and placement needed by each child with a disability to receive FAPE. Children with disabilities have the right to be educated to the maximum extent appropriate in the LRE with children who do not have disabilities. IEP teams must consider a continuum of options to meet each individual child's needs. If a parent does not believe the LEA is providing FAPE for their child, they can invoke their due process rights and DPI and/or a court would consider the applicable facts and make conclusions.

The virtual provision of therapies and other health services has broad implications and that have not yet been resolved from educational, legal, ethical and other licensing-related perspectives.

Collaboration in School for Children without Disabilities

School-based OTs and PTs may have roles in the school setting outside of the special education spectrum. These roles are at the universal level, such as team teaching and providing professional development. The Occupational Therapy Practice Framework identifies five categories of intervention (AOTA 2008), one of which is to create or promote. Depending on the job description, this approach may be an incidental or optional category of occupational therapy intervention in schools, as it is not specific to individuals with disabilities. An OT may provide services that are likely to improve occupational performance for all students in a school. In educational terminology, this approach is often called a universal intervention. Examples include consulting on an ergonomic seating plan, contributing to the design of a playground, developing a backpack awareness program, mentoring teachers in a cognitive-sensory program for self-regulation, and assisting in the development of a schoolwide handwriting curriculum. Hanft and Shepherd (2008) call this approach *system support* and describe it as "an opportunity to apply one's professional wisdom and experience to develop programs and policies to build the capacity of a school district and its education teams."

School-based occupational therapists and physical therapists may have roles in the school setting at the universal level, such as team teaching and providing professional development.

Similarly, a school PT may provide services at the universal level. The PT may also consult on ergonomic seating, help develop backpack programs, and contribute to playground design. In addition, the PT may provide prevention, fitness, and wellness activities as part of universally designed programs for all students. The PT may collaborate with the physical education instructor to adapt the gym environment, equipment, or curriculum so that students with varying levels of strength, stamina, and endurance are able to participate in wellness and fitness activities.

Response to Intervention (RtI)

School district personnel frequently request the participation of OTs and PTs on general education student assistance teams, or *RtI* processes for children not identified with disabilities. Part of the widespread confusion about Response to Intervention (RtI) is that the term is being used to describe a comprehensive, systematic process that is more correctly called Coordinated Early Intervening Services or CEIS. CEIS is general education. DPI's long standing interpretation of state law regarding licensure and funding is that a person holding a special education license may not provide primary instruction, including CEIS, to children who have not been identified as having a disability. Special education teachers may provide support to general education teachers in the form of team teaching, coaching, mentoring, support to regular education teams and professional development. This perspective of providing universal support with school and teachers as *client* is also recommended for OT and PT roles in CEIS. A therapist observing a child in the classroom or participating in student assistance teams and offering intervention strategies for an individual child is not RtI.

This perspective of providing universal support with school and teachers as client is also recommended for occupational therapists and physical therapists.

RtI is defined by Batsche et al. (2005) as the practice of (1) providing high-quality instruction/intervention matched to student needs, and (2) using learning rate over time and level of performance to make important education decisions. RtI in IDEA is specifically tied to eligibility for the category of Specific Learning Disability, although the concept is useful for all children. The idea of RtI is that educators should measure objectively over time a child's response to whatever intervention is used to help him learn. This process is sometimes called progress monitoring. When a general education teacher tries an intervention with a student, she should take data on how it works so that she knows whether to continue it or try something else. Special education teachers, OTs, and PTs working with students who have IEPs should also base their continuation or discontinuation of an intervention on progress monitoring data about the child's response to the intervention.

Screening

Screening, as used in 30 CFR 300.302 and section 614(a)(1)(E) of IDEA refers to a process that a teacher or specialist uses to determine appropriate instructional strategies. Screening is typically a relatively simple and quick process that can be used with groups of children. The term, *instructional strategies for curriculum implementation* is generally used to refer to strategies a teacher may use to teach children more effectively. (Federal Register 2006) Screening is an activity that includes all children in a school, grade or class. Other examples include pre-kindergarten screening, vision screening and hearing screening. Typically, public notice is given offering the screening to the target group. Prior written notice and informed parental consent are not required. OTs and PTs may collaborate with teachers to provide a universal screening to a population of children, such as all preschoolers being screened for kindergarten.

When teachers or other school personnel ask an OT or PT to screen an individual child, they typically are asking the therapist

- to observe a child with an IEP to see if an occupational therapy or physical therapy evaluation is needed.

- to observe a child without an IEP to see if occupational therapy or physical therapy should be part of a special education evaluation.

- to observe a child without an IEP in order to provide child-specific recommendations to the teacher.

OTs and PTs should not observe or screen an individual student who has not been referred for a special education evaluation that includes the respective therapist on the IEP team. PI 11.24 (2) of the Wis. Admin Code reads,

> If a child is suspected to need occupational therapy or physical therapy or both, the IEP team for that child shall include an appropriate therapist.

An OT or PT who intentionally observes or screens a child without formally being part of an IEP team evaluation is making a decision about the child's need for services, based on a limited evaluation. That decision belongs to the child's IEP team, not the therapist alone. If teachers need help knowing what services to recommend to the IEP team, or help in understanding the role of therapy, that information may be provided to them in other ways such as those described later in this chapter.

Since IDEA 1997 and again since IDEA 2004, DPI has advised that adding occupational therapy or physical therapy to a student's IEP requires an initial evaluation or reevaluation. Occupational therapy and physical therapy are regulated not only by special education law, but also by state professional practice acts and licensing standards. These requirements and standards apply to all settings, including school-based practice. Because of these regulations, the school district must initiate a reevaluation process, including notice of reevaluation, review of existing information, decision on testing, and parental consent, if a child with an IEP is suspected to need occupational therapy or physical therapy. They are unique in this respect; other services can be added at an IEP meeting without going through reevaluation.

The parent of a child with an IEP is entitled to certain procedural safeguards described in law. Creating a special consent form does not negate that entitlement. Parents could claim that the school did not provide them with proper

If a child is suspected to need occupational therapy or physical therapy or both, the IEP team for that child shall include an appropriate therapist.

notices of reevaluation, or opportunities to participate in all meetings about their children's FAPE, or notices of options the school considered but rejected.

Serving Students Who Do Not Have IEPs

If a school district decides to provide occupational therapy or physical therapy that is targeted to individual students outside of the IEP team or Section 504 processes, it should do so with a full understanding of its commitment. All licensed occupational therapy practitioners in the state must follow the state occupational therapy licensing and practice rules in the Wisconsin Administrative code (OT 1 through 5). All licensed physical therapy practitioners in the state must follow the state physical therapy licensing and practice rules in the Wisconsin Administrative Code (PT 1 through 9). Chapter PI 11, Wis. Admin Code makes it clear that the intent of allowing schools to provide occupational therapy and physical therapy is to serve children with disabilities. If a school wants to provide targeted occupational therapy or physical therapy to children outside of the IDEA or 504 processes, the school should consider

- licensure rules that require an evaluation that complies with standards of practice prior to providing service.

- licensure rules that require physician referral except for children served under IDEA and Section 504.

- parental informed consent for services to children.

- the possibility of an IDEA complaint that the district conducted an evaluation or made placement without the proper notices and procedures.

- the decision to provide therapy to children without IEPs who break bones, have surgery, need rehabilitation or sensory integration or other clinical services.

- limitations on the use of state categorical aid, federal flow-through funds, and Medicaid funds for occupational therapy and physical therapy that are not driven by IEPs.

Collaboration to Build the Capacity of Teachers

While the overall purpose of the sample checklists in chapter 3, Figures 6 and 7 is to help teachers make appropriate referrals, therapists can gather information from a number of these to customize professional development for a specific group of teachers. Examples are giving an in-service to elementary teachers on teaching handwriting, offering classroom kits for simple accommodations, setting up kindergarten sensory centers, developing movement activities for breaks between academic tasks, and optimizing positioning. By providing support at the universal level to teachers as the *client,* therapists help build the capacity of general educators to work with diverse student needs. In addition to professional development, therapists may also provide support to special education teachers

By providing support at the universal level to teachers as the client, therapists help build the capacity of general educators to work with diverse student needs.

and general education teachers in the form of team teaching, coaching, and mentoring. If the therapist co-teaches a class with the general education teacher and the teacher is present at all times, the therapist may lead the actual instruction as long as she is working with an entire population and not singling out one or a few students.

System Consultation

Educators often possess little information about physical therapy and occupational therapy. Teachers and therapists are educated to assess and emphasize different components of learning, child development, and behavior. They use different terminology and employ different strategies and techniques. Ideally, the principal arranges a short in-service on the roles of the OT and the PT for school staff at the beginning of the school year. The in-service may occur in conjunction with other training or as a separate program, but should include all staff. This meeting includes

- the legal definitions that relate to school therapy.

- the difference between school therapy and clinical therapy.

- the differing roles of occupational therapy and physical therapy.

- the roles of the therapist and therapy assistant.

- the referral process (described in chapter 3).

Therapists may provide the information for the staff in writing, using generally understood terms for later reference. This type of meeting will help to dispel the perceived mystique of the role of the therapist. Once teachers understand the process and benefits of therapy, their support and involvement will increase.

Topical in-services should include a verbal and written explanation of common therapy terms that are related to the school setting.

When there are children within the building who are unable to assume and maintain functional positions due to a disability and who need someone to position them, it is important to provide this training as soon as possible to those responsible for therapeutic positioning, for the health and safety of both the child and the staff. If children require significant assistance in feeding or toileting, training in these areas should also take place early in the school year. Later in the school year, a therapist could provide an in-service on positioning, handwriting, or other subject of frequent consultation requests or referrals. Topical in-services should include a verbal and written explanation of common therapy terms that are related to the school setting.

System consultation also occurs when OTs or PTs assist a school district in making systemwide changes. For instance, therapists may contribute to planning playgrounds or other facilities that are accessible to children with disabilities. They may help design kindergarten screening programs that general educators conduct. System consultation uses the expertise and experience of the therapists to benefit the entire building or district.

Collaboration with Providers Outside of School Environments

Parents, administrators, physicians, and third-party payers struggle to understand the differences between school-based and community-based therapy and how each offers unique services for a child. Knowing the framework in which these two provider groups practice will help families, medical providers, and third-party payers to coordinate services for children. School-based therapy is provided to assist a child with a disability to benefit from special education and is provided only if the child needs therapy to function in the educational setting. Intervention may or may not be provided directly with the child present. Collaborating with educational staff to modify the environment and school routines is always a part of school therapy. School-based therapy is not an outpatient clinic therapy, so interventions such as physical agents or electrotherapeutic modalities are typically not provided. In contrast, the goal of community or clinic-based services is to optimize the child's functional performance in relation to needs in home and community settings. Therapy usually occurs in a hospital, rehabilitation facility, outpatient clinic, or the child's home and may involve a greater array of services and modalities not ordinarily needed in a school setting. The therapist typically works with the child individually. Therapy might include post-surgical intervention, soft tissue mobilization, joint mobilization, self-care training, or a specialty technique.

Sometimes the objectives of school-based therapy may be identical to the objectives of community-based therapy. The child may have educationally related needs that also occur in other environments. For instance, following surgery, a student with an orthopedic impairment may receive school-based physical therapy to enable the student to walk between classrooms and other locations in school. A clinical PT may do similar interventions with the same child for strength, flexibility, endurance, speed, or accuracy of movement in the home or community environments.

Conversely, the objectives in the community-based therapy may be unrelated or complementary to the objectives in school-based therapy. For example, a young student with a learning disability may receive occupational therapy in school to enable her to regulate responses to sensory aspects of the school environment. A community-based OT may work with the same child at the family's home in developing self-care routines and organizational strategies. The interventions used in both settings may be similar or different. It is good practice, and a requirement of some third-party payers, for the school-based therapist and the community-based therapist to communicate and plan a child's therapy together. Collaboration between the school and community therapists is essential to coordinate the child's therapy and prevent duplication of services. Collaboration may take the form of phone calls, e-mails, participation in a hospital staffing, or IEP meetings.

The objectives in community-based therapy may be related, unrelated or complementary to the objectives in school-based therapy.

Collaboration with Parents

IDEA emphasizes that schools and parents have a shared responsibility in educating students. The law grants certain rights to students and their parents that schools must observe in the special education process: research shows that a positive relationship among all partners is crucial to student success. It just makes sense to establish effective two-way communication between parents and school personnel, provide parents with accurate information about the IEP team process and services, and place an emphasis on relationships with parents as collaborative decision makers. Schools and educational staff must take the lead to facilitate the involvement of families, recognizing that all families have strengths and care about their child's well-being.

Communication

When a child is referred for an IEP team evaluation, parents' opinions and observations are critical, and educators and therapists must respect and value them. The inclusion of information from the child's parents in the evaluation data helps to ensure that everyone has the same understanding of the child. Parents often bring information from previous evaluations and interventions, as well as knowledge of their child's personality, preferences and accomplishments.

It just makes sense to establish effective two-way communication between parents and school personnel.

An exchange of information will most often take place during the IEP team meeting. It is important that this is a true exchange among the parent, therapist, and teachers in order for the team members to design a program that will be of real benefit to the child. Parents' questions need to be answered in generally understandable terms, so that they will continue to be comfortable asking questions during the school years.

Sometimes parents come to the IEP team meeting with a firm idea of a specific intervention that they want for their child. When teachers or school therapists have different opinions, conflict may arise. Conflict is a natural consequence of bringing together diverse perspectives. Differences in thinking increase the likelihood of more creative solutions for students. To approach conflict positively and successfully, team members must try to articulate their underlying interests and probe the opposing perspective to find out if there is a solution that can integrate the interests of all. When team members respond effectively to the presence of conflict, it can lead to improved understanding, stronger relationships, and more effective problem solving. The DPI website page on *Creating Agreement* offers resources for school personnel and families to learn about positive conflict resolution.

During the course of actual therapy, it is a priority for each therapist involved with a child and his or her family to establish clear communication. Methods of communication with parents may include a home-to-school notebook, telephone calls, e-mails, or online social networking. Positive messages that share the child's strengths and progress can strengthen relationships with parents.

Accurate Information

When a child is referred to special education for the first time, his parent may need an explanation of the IEP team process and a discussion of the role of the parent as an important IEP team member. In addition to the Procedural Safeguards notice required by law, parents should be given accurate, understandable information. Most school districts, as well as DPI, the Wisconsin Statewide Parent-Educator Initiative, and Wisconsin FACETS can provide parents with free, accurate resources in various languages and media forms to explain the complexities of the IEP team process.

Specific to school- based therapy, parents may benefit from an explanation of service delivery models, the process of assigning therapists, and a description of school-based and community-based therapy. Parents must understand the difference between family centered, community-based therapy, and related services. If their opinions and questions about school-based therapy receive attention and respect, their expectations of therapy as a related service to education will become differentiated from their experiences with clinical therapy. When the services on the child's IEP are integrated and service providers operate as a team, it is easier for a parent to understand that the child's individual program will vary from year to year, as the child's needs change. Therapy may be more frequent for a younger child who is learning play skills or writing, than for a child at the middle school level who has begun to change classes and adjust to a new environment. Therapy may fit into an older child's schedule in a different way than it does for the younger child. At the high school level, the student's therapy is directed toward preparation for post-high school educational and vocational goals and adult living arrangements. In any given year, a student's occupational therapy and physical therapy may increase or decrease, be discontinued or be resumed, based on the goals in the student's IEP. When this is understood by all from the very first IEP meeting, the participants are more likely to agree upon subsequent decisions about occupational therapy and physical therapy.

Shared Decision Making

As a way to ensure that parents are equal team members, the school may provide an IEP worksheet for the parents to fill out and bring to the IEP meeting. Other tools such as a written agenda for the IEP team meeting, staff contact information, and a file folder for the parent's copies of records can help the parent participate more knowledgeably and comfortably on the team. Staff can also share with parents the contact information for the parent liaison, district parent resources, and state resources. Parents who feel they are a part of planning the child's program are better able to understand how their child will benefit and may be able to complement the program at home. Parents can be effective members of the intervention team through activities at home if they have adequate information and training in the process. Therapists should be cautious about imposing home program expectations, but some parents will welcome suggestions.

A written agenda for the IEP team meeting, staff contact information, and a file folder for the parent's copies of records can help the parent participate.

The student takes part in decision-making about his or her program, and at the age of eighteen, legally assumes the responsibility that once belonged to the parent. In Wisconsin, a student must be invited to the IEP team meeting if he or she will be fourteen years of age or older during the time that the new IEP will be in effect. In most instances, it is beneficial for the student to attend at least part the meeting at younger ages, to become comfortable with the process of self-determination and self-advocacy.

Procedural Safeguards

IDEA requires schools to provide parents of a child with a disability with a notice containing a full explanation of the procedural safeguards available under the IDEA and U.S. Department of Education regulations. The complete text of the notice is available on the DPI website. School therapists should be aware of the following rights and procedural safeguards that parents and adult students have under the law.

- The school must tell parents in writing what it plans to do, or refuses to do, before it does it, and why. This includes when a school

  — proposes to initiate or to change the identification, evaluation, or educational placement of the child, or the provision of FAPE to the child.

  — refuses to initiate or to change the identification, evaluation, or educational placement of the child, or the provision of FAPE to the child.

- Parents have the right to participate in all meetings that the school holds about the above actions.

- Parental consent is needed before school personnel may conduct any assessment in an evaluation or reevaluation, provide special education for the first time, or release confidential records. Parents may withdraw consent for an evaluation or reevaluation that is in process but the withdrawal is not retroactive. Parents may revoke consent for the provision of all special education and related services but they may not select some services and not others.

- Consent means a parent is fully informed in his or her native language, understands the proposed action and voluntarily agrees in writing to the described activity.

- Parents have the right to review all educational records of their child.

- When parents disagree with the results of an evaluation, they may obtain an Independent Educational Evaluation at the expense of the school district.

School therapists should be aware of the rights and procedural safeguards that parents and adult students have under the law.

- When parents disagree with an action of the school or believe that special education law has been violated, they have a right to file a State Complaint, request mediation, and/or request a due process hearing.

- Parents have certain protections when a school disciplines a child with a disability.

- Parents have limited access to public school services when they place their children in private schools.

Homeless Children and Out-of-State Transfer

The rights of homeless children came to the forefront with Hurricane Katrina in 2005. Under the McKinney-Vento Act, homeless students have a right to enroll in school and to receive all public school services, including special education and related services. To comply with IDEA 2004, districts must provide children with disabilities with a FAPE when they enroll in the district from out of state.

Schools must enroll students who are relocating to the school district immediately. If the district does not have the student's records, the district shall take reasonable steps to obtain promptly the records from the student's previous school. Such records include the IEP and supporting documents and any other records relating to the provision of special education or related services.

The district shall initiate special education services without delay. If a parent is available, district staff consults with the parent prior to initiating special education services. The district should not require written parental consent as a condition for providing special education services to transfer students from out of state. The parent already consented to the provision of special education and related services in the state of origin.

Before providing occupational therapy, the OT must have medical information about the child. The amount of medical information the OT needs to ensure the child's safety depends on the child's medical history. Reviewing existing data in the out-of-state IEP and other pupil records may provide the medical information the OT needs. Information also may be obtained from the parent, patient health care provider including out-of-state medical providers, or other reliable source.

A PT must have medical information from a licensed physician regarding a child before the child receives physical therapy. The information may come from a licensed physician in the state of origin or from a local physician. Existing data in the child's out-of-state IEP or other pupil records may include information from a licensed physician. When this information is unavailable, an examination by a local licensed physician is required. The district must ensure it is obtained at no cost to the parent.

Culturally Responsive Education

Students in Wisconsin schools today vary in culture, language, abilities, and many other characteristics. For many students, the kinds of behaviors that school requires and the way that school staff communicates contrast with cultural and

---

Each teacher and therapist has a responsibility to engage in personal processes to become culturally responsive.

language practices at home. (Richards et al. 2007) By recognizing and using students' strengths, school therapists engage in culturally responsive education to facilitate the achievement of all students.

Every student has the ability to learn, yet schools struggle to effectively educate all students. Administrative policies and practices of the school are important to establishing an environment of cultural responsiveness, but each teacher and therapist has a responsibility to engage in personal processes to become culturally responsive. Too often, race is a predictor of success in Wisconsin schools. (DPI 2008) Where research has revealed likely contributing factors, rarely are intentional actions or blatant incidents of discrimination identified as the cause of the racial disparities in special education. Research does suggest, however, that far more subtle and unconscious forms of race, gender and class bias may contribute to disparities. Awareness is key. Research also indicates that the racial disparities in special education are the result of shared challenges in both special and general education. Some specific approaches to a personal process of increasing cultural competency are available on the website for "Culturally Responsive Education for All: Training and Enhancement" (www.createwisconsin.net). Both AOTA and APTA have resources related to cultural competency for OTs and PTs.

Another component of culturally responsive education, the instructional dimension, includes materials, strategies, and activities that form the basis of instruction or intervention. These include guidelines such as

- acknowledging students' differences as well as their commonalities.

- validating students' cultural identity in classroom practices and instructional materials.

- assessing students' ability and achievement validly.

- fostering a positive interrelationship among students, their families, the community, and school.

- motivating students to become active participants in their learning. (Richards et al. 2007)

Culturally responsive education is essential to effective interactions with students and families, and it affects student outcomes. When culturally responsive education is in place, all school staff welcome and support all students, regardless of their language and cultural background.

References

American Academy of Pediatrics. 2008. "School Bus Transportation of Children with Special Health Care Needs." http://aappolicy.aappublications.org/cgi/content/full/pediatrics;108/2/516 (accessed August 11, 2010).

American Academy of Pediatrics. 2010. *Car Safety Seats: A Guide for Families.* http://www.aap.org/family/carseatguide.htm (accessed August 11, 2010).

American Occupational Therapy Association (AOTA). 2008. "Occupational Therapy Practice Framework: Domain and Process Second Edition." *American Journal of Occupational Therapy* 62: 25-683.

Batsche, G., J. Elliott, J. Graden, J. Grimes, J. Kovaleski, D. Prasse, D. Reschly, J. Schrag and W. Tilly. 2005. *Response to Intervention: Policy Considerations and Implementation.* Alexandria, VA: National Association of State Directors of Special Education, Inc. 5-6.

Darragh, A. and E. and Hussey. 2008. "Safe Movement and Handling Methods: Application in the School Setting." Presentation at the Statewide School Based OT and PT Conference, Wisconsin Dells, WI.

Federal Register 71(156): 46639. Monday, August 14, 2006.

Hanft, B. and P. Place. 1996. *The Consulting Therapist: A Guide for OTs and PTs in Schools.* San Antonio: Pearson Education, Inc.

Hanft, B. & J. Shepard. 2008. *Collaborating for Student Success: A Guide for School-Based Occupational Therapy.* Bethesda, MD: AOTA Press.

Health Resources and Services Administration, U.S. Department of Health and Human Services. 2010. "Telehealth." http://www.hrsa.gov/telehealth/default.htm (accessed August 11, 2010).

Kaminker, M., L. Chiarello, and J. Chiarini Smith. 2006. "Decision Making for Physical Therapy Service Delivery in Schools: A Nationwide Analysis by Geographic Region." *Pediatric Physical Therapy* 18(3): 204-213.

McWilliam, R.A. 2010. *Routines-Based Early Intervention: Supporting Young Children and Their Families.* Baltimore: Paul H. Brookes Publishing Co., Inc.

___. 1995. "Integration of therapy and consultative special education: A continuum in early intervention." *Infants and Young Children*, 7(4), 29-38.

National Institute on Disability and Rehabilitation Research, U.S. Dept. of Education. "AbleData." http://abledata.com/abledata.cfm (accessed August 17, 2010)

Kutschera, D. 2009. "Special Education Procedures for Equipment Systems." Neenah Joint School District, Neenah WI.

Occupational Safety and Health Administration. 2009. "Ergonomics for the Prevention of Musculoskeletal Disorders." *Guidelines for Nursing Homes. OSHA 3182-3R.* http://www.osha.gov/ergonomics/guidelines/nursinghome/final_nh_guidelines.pdf (accessed August 11, 2010).

Rainforth, B. and J. York-Barr. 1997. *Collaborative Teams for Students with Severe Disabilities,* 2nd Edition. Baltimore: Paul H. Brookes Publishing Co., Inc. 27.

Rehabilitation Engineering Research Center on Wheelchair Safety and University of Michigan Transportation Research Institute University of Michigan Health System. "Ride Safe." Copyright 2009. http://travelsafer.org/ (accessed March 16, 2010).

Richards, H.V., A. F. Brown, and T. B. Forde. 2007. *Addressing Diversity in Schools: Culturally Responsive Pedagogy.* Tempe, AZ: National Center for Culturally Responsive Educational Systems.

Russell, T.G. 2007. Physical Rehabilitation Using Telemedicine. *Journal of Telemedicine and Telecare* 13: 217-220.

Scheideman-Miller, C. 2004. "Rehabilitation." In J. Tracy, *Telemedicine Technical Assistance Documents: A Guide to Getting Started.* University of Missouri School of Medicine. http://telehealth.muhealth.org/general%20information/getting.started.telemedicine.pdf (accessed August 17, 2010).

Society of Automotive Engineers, Inc. "Wheelchair Tiedowns and Occupant Restraints for Use in Motor Vehicles." 2010. http://www.sae.org/technical/standards/J2249_199901 (accessed March 16, 2010).

Wisconsin Department of Public Instruction. 2008. "Annotated Checklist for Addressing Racial Disproportionality in Special Education." http://www.createwisconsin.net/cms_files/resources/062409onlinechecklist.doc

Other Resources

Heimerl, S., and N. Rasch. 2009, September. Delivering Developmental Occupational Therapy Consultation Services through Telehealth. *Developmental Disabilities Special Interest Section Quarterly* 32(3):1-4. American Occupational Therapy Association.

McWilliam, R.A. and S. Scott. 2003. *Integrating Therapy into the Classroom.* National Individualizing Preschool Inclusion Project, August 2003.

McWilliam, R.A. and A. M. Casey. 2008. *Engagement of Every Child in the Preschool Classroom.* Baltimore: Paul H. Brookes Publishing Co., Inc.

National Highway Traffic Safety Administration (NHTSA). "The Federal Motor Vehicle Safety Standards (FMVSS 222)." www.nhtsa.dot.gov. (accessed March 16, 2010).

Rehabilitation Engineering Research Center (RERC), WC19. "Wheelchairs and Seating Systems successfully crash tested with 4-point strap-type securement as of July 27, 2009."
http://www.rercwts.org/RERC_WTS2_KT/RERC_WTS2_KT_Stand/RERC_WTS2_19_Chart.html (accessed March 16, 2010).

Wisconsin Department of Public Instruction. 2010. "Creating Agreement." http://www.dpi.wi.gov/sped/agreement.html (accessed August 11, 2010).

___. 2010. "Wisconsin Statewide Parent-Educator Initiative, Information Especially for Parents" http://www.dpi.wi.gov/sped/hmparents.html (accessed August 11, 2010).

___. 2009. "Directives for the Use of Seclusion and Physical Restraint in Special Education Programs." http://dpi.wi.gov/sped/sbseclusion.html (accessed August 11, 2010).

___. 2009. "Information Update on Transportation." http://www.dpi.wi.gov/sped/pdf/bul09-02.pdf (accessed August 11, 2010).

___. 2009. "Procedural Safeguards Notice." http://www.dpi.wi.gov/sped/pcrights.html (accessed August 11, 2010).

___. IDEA complaint decisions 07-075, 08-006, and 08-092. http://dpi.wi.gov/sped/com07men.html and http://dpi.wi.gov/sped/com08men.html.

Wisconsin Family Assistance Center for Education, Training and Support http://www.wifacets.org/ (accessed August 11, 2010).

Wisconsin State Patrol. "Wisconsin State Patrol is responsible for bus inspection and has information on Wisconsin regulations and requirements." www.dot.wisconsin.gov/statepatrol (accessed March 16, 2010).

Administration of Occupational Therapy and Physical Therapy in School

8

The administration of occupational therapy and physical therapy is typically the responsibility of the director of special education. In some districts, the district administrator takes this responsibility. The director oversees the employment and supervision of therapy staff, budget preparation, implementation of IEPs and accountability for the provision of related services. Administration of related services includes determining the school district's need for occupational therapy and physical therapy staff; providing staff; assuring quality service provision; and obtaining funding for related services.

Determining Service Need

The term *service need* refers to the total amount of time a district needs from therapy personnel. The following factors determine the service need for each of the related services of occupational therapy and physical therapy.

- the amounts of occupational therapy or physical therapy on all the children's IEPs

- the caseload of each therapist

- the workload of each therapist

- contractual guarantees stipulated by a master agreement

Descriptions of the components of service need follow. Examples of how the special education director may calculate these amounts of time are shown in Figure 27 on the following page.

Amount of Service on IEPs

A school district provides occupational therapy and physical therapy to a child with a disability when that child requires those services to benefit from special education. The IEP team makes this determination. Therapy may be direct or indirect, and provided individually or in a group. The IEP team decides the amount, frequency, duration, and location of a specific related service the district will provide, and records that information on the IEP. The amount and frequency of occupational therapy or physical therapy service is stated on the IEP

Therapy may be direct or indirect, and provided individually or in a group.

Figure 27 Sample Occupational Therapy Annual Projection

Student	Frequency and minutes per session				Current building
	Direct		Indirect		
A.M.	1x/week	45	1x/week	15	West
B.K.	2x/week	30	1x/week	15	King
B.S.	2x/week	45	1x/week	15	South
B.J.	2x/week	30	1x/week	15	East
B.C.	1x/semester	30	1x/week	15	King
B. T.	2x/week	30	1x/week	15	Kennedy
D.K.	1x/week	30	1x/week	15	Kennedy
D.A.	2x/week	30	1x/week	15	East
E.J.	2x/week	30	1x/week	15	King
H.K.	1x/week	45	1x/week	15	South
K.N.	2x/week	45	1x/week	15	South
K.S.	Moved				Kennedy
K.E.	2x/week	group:	1x/week	15	King
M.A.	2x/week	45	1x/week	15	Kennedy
M.T.	2x/week		1x/week	15	North
M.S.	Expect to discontinue				North
M.B.			2x/semester	60	North
M.D.			1x/month	45	Kennedy
N.A.			1x/month	30	King
R.V.	2x/week	30	1x/week	15	King
R.D.	2x/week	30	1x/week	15	King
S.D.	2x/week	30	1x/week	15	Kennedy
S.B.			1x/month	30	East
S.J.	2x/week	30	1x/week	15	West
S.A.	1x/week	45	1x/week	15	West
S.T.	2x/week	30	1x/week	15	North
T.B.	2x/week	30	1x/week	15	Kennedy
T.D.	Expect to discontinue				King
T.M.	2x/week	30	1x/week	15	King
W.M.		30	1x/quarter	30	Kennedy

30 Students 19.25 hours per week 6.0 hours per week 6 buildings

Average Weekly Totals:
25.25 hours direct and indirect services
 5.75 hours travel, set-up, and exit
 2.0 hours evaluations, IEP team meetings, staff meeting
 4.0 hours evaluation reports, treatment plans, progress notes, Medicaid documentation
 <u>3.0 hours anticipated growth in caseload</u>
40 hours weekly occupational therapy service

Program Summary Page and can be found in the section on related services, supplementary aids and services, or program modifications or supports for school personnel. The director adds the number of hours or minutes of occupational therapy or physical therapy that all the IEPs document to determine the total time a district requires for direct or indirect therapy to children and supports for school personnel.

Caseload

Caseload requirements for occupational therapists (OTs) and physical therapists (PTs) are in Chapter PI 11.24, Wis. Admin Code. The minimum caseload for a full-time therapist is 15 students. The maximum caseload for a full-time therapist is 30 students, but with a licensed assistant(s) can reach 45 students. Caseload is prorated for part-time therapists. Chapter PI 11, Wis. Admin Code allows for variance among the numbers based on several identified factors. These include the frequency and duration of the service listed on the child's IEP, travel time, evaluations, preparation, and other student-related activities. Students receiving indirect service or consultation are considered part of the therapist's caseload. Indirect service, collaborative consultation, and coaching are methods of service delivery that support the student's participation in the general education curriculum and educational environment. These three—indirect service, collaborative consultation, or coaching—may take as much or more time than direct service.

Experience has shown that when therapy caseloads exceed the maximum, problems occur.

Experience has shown that when therapy caseloads exceed the maximum, problems occur in meeting the amount and frequency of therapy in students' IEPs; therapist retention becomes an issue; caseload adjustments are made for administrative convenience; and parental complaints increase. As part of the State Superintendent's Task Force on Caseloads in Special Education, researchers at the University of Wisconsin (UW)-Oshkosh conducted a study entitled *Occupational and Physical Therapy Caseload Size: Service Provision and Perceptions of Efficacy* (Chiang and Rylance, 2000) The study found that full-time therapists serve an average of 32 students and full-time therapists with assistants serve 43 students. Although these numbers indicate that the average therapist is working at or near the maximum caseload capacity, caseload numbers alone do not capture the complexity of school-based therapists' work.

Workload

In the article, *Transforming Caseload to Workload in School-Based and Early Intervention Occupational Therapy Services,* the American Occupational Therapy Association (AOTA) recommends using the term *workload* rather than *caseload* for school-based practice. (AOTA 2006) *Workload* encompasses all of the work activities that therapists perform that benefit students directly and indirectly. Workload includes

- providing direct therapy services and interventions.

- consulting, coaching or collaborating with others to integrate therapy into classroom and school activities.

- conducting evaluations of children.

- collecting and analyzing data on the effectiveness of interventions.

- attending IEP team and other meetings.

- preparing written reports to meet school district and license requirements.

- preparing or securing materials and adaptive equipment.

- communicating with other agencies, therapists, physicians, parents, and school staff.

- providing therapy required by Section 504 plans.

- traveling between sites.

- supervising assistants.

- training staff and parents.

- participating in school-wide activities.

- performing other assigned tasks.

The therapist reviews time study data and calculates the percentage of time spent performing each activity.

Workload management begins with completing a time study that includes all the child-related activities and tasks the therapist performs. The therapist develops a weekly or monthly workload table with 15 or 30 minute time slots for the following: student therapy sessions that IEPs require, collaboration with other staff, new evaluations, contacts with community providers, meetings, paperwork, travel, supervision, and lunch. The therapist reviews this time study data and calculates the percentage of time spent performing each activity. The therapist and the administrator then can analyze the demands of the therapist's workload.

The Pediatric Section of the American Physical Therapy Association (APTA) has a School-Based Special Interest Group with a Workload Subcommittee for School-Based Physical Therapists. Members of the workgroup completed time studies and their findings support the AOTA workload concept. (Cecere 2008) Both OTs and PTs carry a significant and varied workload. Some of the descriptive statistics from the workload study appear here.

"Overall percentages of time spent in each category:

- Direct: 40%

- Indirect: 11.63%

- Meetings: 2.1%

- Program documentation (daily notes): 18.63%

- Travel: 10.18%

- Professional development: 3.2%

- Supervision and mentoring: 3.7%

- IEP documentation: 6.6%

- Pre-intervening: 3.3%

- Other: 10.55%

The time pattern was spent on an average of 21.95 students by PTs with 11.62 years of experience." (Cecere 2010, 5)

Travel

Travel is a therapy-related activity that may include packing and loading materials and equipment, traveling the distance to the next site, unloading and unpacking materials and equipment, and setting up for services. Adequate travel time between schools or other sites varies depending on the distance, the individual needs of the children, the availability of materials and equipment in multiple sites, road conditions, and weather conditions.

Documentation

Documentation of occupational therapy and physical therapy is both a legal requirement and a means of evaluating a child's response to intervention. Adequate documentation is essential for third-party reimbursement of services, substantiation of the delivery of service, and assessment of the effectiveness of service management. Service need includes time for therapists to

- obtain medical information.

- document evaluation results.

- prepare for IEP meetings.

- develop and revise treatment or intervention plans.

- maintain regular attendance records.

- update progress notes, including specialized documentation required for third-party billing and data collection on IEP goals.

- write occupational therapy and physical therapy discontinuance reports.

- record supervision meetings with occupational therapy assistants (OTAs) and physical therapist assistants (PTAs).

- prepare statistical records and reports required for administrative functions.

- maintain records related to supplies and equipment.

- prepare other documentation that the school districts or practice regulations require.

Supervision

When a district employs OTAs or PTAs, the director must allocate time for therapists to supervise the assistants. Supervision requirements are found in Chapter PI 11.24, Wis. Admin Code and the professional practice regulations as discussed in chapter 6.

Documentation is both a legal requirement and a means of evaluating a child's response to intervention.

Contractual Guarantees

Therapists hired under teacher contracts by the school district have working condition stipulations in accordance with the master agreement. These stipulations may include opportunities for staff meetings, continuing education days, visitations, duty-free lunches, length of day, and student contact provisions. The director of special education must incorporate these factors into the determination of service need.

Providing Staff

As noted in chapter 6, a critical shortage of OTs and PTs existed in Wisconsin in the 1990s. Despite a brief respite from this shortage, it appears to have returned, and the data collected about its patterns and causes may prove helpful here. The Wisconsin Educator Supply and Demand Project conducted a 1995 Related Services survey, to which 93 percent of Wisconsin school districts and CESAs responded. The responses indicated that

- 29 percent of respondents required six months or more to fill a PT position.

- 18 percent of respondents required six months or more to fill an OT position.

- 61 percent of respondents had only one applicant for a PT position.

- 32 percent of respondents had only one applicant for an OT position.

The availability of OTs and PTs varies within the state. The survey results suggest that in areas of low availability, school districts must begin recruiting more than six months in advance of the date staff are needed, and may have a limited choice of applicants.

CESA 1 also conducted a survey in 1995, contacting over 5,000 OTs and PTs certified or licensed to practice in Wisconsin. Although the responses varied by CESA, some of the top factors that therapists reported would influence their decision to work in schools were

- the therapist's ability to work with certain student populations, and related needs for retraining.

- a supportive team environment and strong administrative support.

- a competitive salary and benefits.

- the flexible schedule and attractive vacation time typical of school calendars.

- the availability of office space and adequate time for documentation.

In the late 1990s, events occurred that contributed to an increase in the supply of school-based therapists and assistants and the shortage seemed to subside. Changes in federal legislation affected Medicare and Medicaid programs and led to a decrease in demand for therapists and assistants in medical and health care settings. There was also an increase in therapy training programs and an expansion of the number of students accepted into training programs. The shortage however, appears to be resurfacing. The Wisconsin Educator Supply and Demand Project (DPI 2006) states that the supply rating for OT and PT is in the below average range with a ratio of applicants to vacancies at 2.93. A 2007 study by APTA of acute care hospitals found the vacancy rate for PTs was 13.8 percent and for PTAs was 12 percent. The turnover rate for full-time PTs was 15.9 percent and for full-time PTAs was 12.5 percent. The APTA also provides a demographic description of its members. The demographic profile (1999-2006) shows that only 4.2 percent of the PTs and only 2.5 percent of PTAs work in school systems. (APTA 2008) The Center on Personnel Studies in Special Education (COPSSE) noted that nationwide there is a growing shortage of qualified school-based related service personnel. (COPSSE 2004) COPSSE further reports that there has been and continues to be a shortage of qualified PTs in the schools with most shortages in rural areas. COPSSE also reported a shortage of OTs. Factors that contribute to the shortage of school-based OTs are the declining enrollments in occupational therapy training programs, a decrease of 37 percent from 1999-2002; and declining interest in school-based practice as a graduate's first employment choice. According to the 2008-09 *Occupational Outlook Handbook* from the Bureau of Labor Statistics, between 2006 and 2016 the expected increase in employment of OTs is 23 percent; of OTAs is 25 percent; of PTs is 27 percent; and of PTAs is 32 percent. Growth in these professions is much faster than the average for all occupations.

A critical shortage of OTs and PTs existed in Wisconsin in the 1990s. Despite a brief respite from this shortage, it appears to have returned.

Recruitment

School districts use a variety of approaches to locate OTs and PTs for employment. Appendix F contains sample position descriptions for a school OT, school PT, school OTA and school PTA. Directors can post vacancies on these online employment sites that are also listed in the references at the end of this chapter:

- Wisconsin educator jobs.

- Wisconsin Education Career Access Network (WECAN).

- Wisconsin Occupational Therapy Association (WOTA) and Wisconsin Physical Therapy Association (WPTA) newsletters.

- School Therapy newsletter that is archived online at cesa1.k12.wi.us.

Other options that directors report as successful in recruiting candidates include

- contacting professional education programs in Wisconsin and neighboring states.

- contacting Regional Service Network directors for information on recruitment projects and mailing lists of Wisconsin therapists within the CESA.

- asking a therapist to post a printed advertisement on a job board at WOTA or WPTA meetings, conferences, and workshops.

- contacting CESA offices, hospitals, public agencies, and private agencies for purchase-of-service agreements.

- contacting parents who might be obtaining private therapy and offering that therapist a contract.

School districts may find it necessary to establish short-term contracts with several individuals or agencies.

Directors may wish to consider an ongoing and proactive approach to filling staff vacancies and anticipating increased service needs. This includes offering district-, or CESA-sponsored continuing education workshops to an established contact list of therapists who are not presently employed by the district; offering a school-based colleague as a mentor to a therapist whose experience is outside of school-based practice; offering fieldwork sites and clinical internships to students in occupational therapy and physical therapy programs at universities and technical colleges; and recruiting at least six months in advance of a vacancy.

When vacancies occur unexpectedly or are prolonged, directors must make every effort to provide children with the therapy that is on their IEPs. School districts may find it necessary to establish short-term contracts with several individuals or agencies to meet these requirements. Directors should notify parents of the situation and enlist their help in finding therapists. Figure 28 on the next page is a sample letter a district sent to parents when an unanticipated vacancy occurred in physical therapy.

Salary

Districts pay therapists and assistants in different ways depending on how the therapist or assistant is employed. A UW-Oshkosh research study found that 65 percent of OTs were employed directly by school systems and 35 percent by service agencies, while 56 percent of PTs were employed directly by school systems and 44 percent by service agencies. When a district hires the therapist or assistant directly, the district may calculate the therapist's salary based upon the teacher salary schedule. In some districts, therapists and assistants are part of the union, and contractual agreements determine wages and benefits. When a district contracts with a CESA, hospital or private agency for therapy services, the contract specifies the amount the district pays for services, but the CESA, hospital, or private agency pays the therapist's or assistant's salary. The DPI Data Management Reporting Team provides position analysis summaries based on the

Figure 28 Sample Parent Letter for Unanticipated Therapist Vacancy

(School Letterhead)

(Date)
(Inside address)
Dear (salutation):

Your child, (name of child), (DOB), has physical therapy services identified in his/her current IEP. The (district) School District has been unable to hire a qualified physical therapist to fill the vacant position. We continue to search actively for qualified candidates throughout the region. Our efforts have included postings in surrounding state universities, advertisements in Internet job sites and community and area newspapers, and contacts with private agencies for purchase of services. We have also kept the DPI consultant apprised of our situation. This correspondence is to notify you that, due to lack of staff, physical therapy will not be able to be provided for (name of child) at this time. The attached sheet identifies private agencies in the community that provide physical therapy. If you are able to acquire outside services, the district will pay for the cost of this service up to the identified amount and frequency specified on the current IEP. Please do the following in seeking district payment for these services.

1. Contact an outside agency to secure physical therapy services.
2. Request, in writing, that these services be paid for by the (district) Public Schools. This should be sent to (name), Supervisor of Special Education, (address), (city, state, zip). The correspondence should include the agency name and the name of the therapist who will be working with your child. Suggested agencies are listed below, but you are not limited to them, and services at these agencies are subject to availability. Enclose a signed consent to release school records to the agency for the purpose of providing school physical therapy.
3. After receiving your written request, the district will confirm your contact with the agency and write a contract to pay for the amount of physical therapy specified in the child's IEP.
4. This district will then confirm the arrangements with you in writing.
5. When you receive verbal and/or written confirmation from the district, you should contact the agency to set up an appointment schedule for services. If you prefer that the district implement this step, please contact me.

The district will continue earnest efforts to locate services in the area of physical therapy. Please contact me if you have additional questions.

Sincerely,

(Name)
Supervisor of Special Education

cc: (Director of Instruction)
    (Supervisor of Administrative Services)
    (Building Principals)
    (DPI Consultant)

PI-1202 Staff Report. A district may request the position analysis summary for an OT, PT, OTA, or PTA from the department. The report contains low, high, and average salary; average fringe; and average length of experience. To receive this report, districts may contact the team at 608-267-3166 or:

Data Management Reporting Team
Department of Public Instruction
PO Box 7841
Madison, WI 53707-7841

Another source for salary information is the Bureau for Labor Statistics. The website http://www.bls.gov/oes/current/oes_nat.htm#b29-0000 provides therapists' salaries, and http://www.bls.gov/oes/current/oes_nat.htm#b31-0000 provides assistants' salaries. OTs and OTAs who are members of AOTA, and PTs and PTAs who are members of APTA can find current demographic information and reports on median salary incomes for their respective positions on these professional websites.

Education Level

Currently licensed OTs and PTs may have bachelor's, master's or doctoral degrees. Accredited education programs no longer offer a bachelor's degree in either occupational therapy or physical therapy. All Wisconsin physical therapy training programs have changed from a master's degree to the doctor of physical therapy degree (DPT). Some PTs with baccalaureate degrees or master's degrees are pursuing a transitional doctor of physical therapy (tDPT). Others may have or may be pursuing a scientific doctorate in an area other than physical therapy. The APTA offers specialist certification to recognize PTs with advanced clinical practice. Certification is awarded to PTs who successfully complete a standardized application and examination process. A PT may become a certified pediatric clinical specialist by successfully completing this process. The status of *board-certified specialist* is evidence of clinical expertise and excellence, but is not an academic degree. An experienced school-based PT may demonstrate these competencies even though the therapist does not have the certification.

As of 2010, occupational therapy training programs offer master's and doctoral degrees in occupational therapy. Four programs allow a person with a master's degree in another field to pursue a doctorate in occupational therapy. The remaining doctoral programs require a previous degree in occupational therapy. OTs frequently pursue master's and doctoral degrees in other related fields. In addition, the AOTA offers board certification in pediatrics and specialty certification in the areas of driving and community mobility; environmental modification; feeding, eating, and swallowing; and low vision.

A challenge for districts is compensating therapists based upon these various educational levels, clinical specialist certification, and pediatric or school-based experience. Districts find that the master's degree or PhD is compatible with the teacher salary schedule. The DPT is a clinical doctorate so districts may consider whether this correlates with the PhD on the teacher salary schedule.

Accredited education programs no longer offer a bachelor's degree in either occupational therapy or physical therapy.

License renewal through the Department of Regulation and Licensing (DRL) for all OTs, OTAs, PTs, and PTAs requires continuing education that focuses on their profession, and is not limited to university classes or credits. Districts may consider continuing education when they determine salaries.

Career advancement opportunities for therapists in the school system are limited. Experienced therapists can only move into licensed administrative positions if they complete a teacher education program. Some large districts and CESAs have a coordinator position for therapists comparable to a program support teacher.

Contracting Options

School districts may recruit and hire therapists through school contracts or purchase-of-service agreements. School boards may write teacher contracts in accordance with the district's master agreement for therapists hired by an individual district or with other districts through a 66.30 agreement. (Chapter PI 14.02, Wis. Admin Code pursuant to s.66.0301, Wis. Stats.) Contracts may be full-time or part-time.

School boards may contract with private or public agencies for physical therapy or occupational therapy services on the basis of demonstrated need. (s.115.88(1), Wis. Stats.) Purchase-of-service agreements may be with a CESA, an individual therapist, a private hospital, or a private therapy agency. Figure 29 on the following pages is a sample purchase-of-service agreement between a school board and an agency for therapy services. A purchase-of-service agreement includes these features:

School boards may contract with private or public agencies for physical therapy or occupational therapy.

- purpose of the agreement

- guarantee and evidence of appropriate DRL and DPI license of therapist or assistant

- availability of replacement therapists from agency

- working conditions

- documentation expectations of the contracting school district or CESA

- other expectations of the contracting school district or CESA

- identification of supervisory relationships and evaluation of staff performance

- identification of how the parties will resolve identified deficiencies

- payment schedule

- cost of service and travel

- effective dates

- renewal conditions

- liability

Figure 29 Sample Purchase of Service Agreement

This Purchase of Service Agreement (this *Agreement*) is made effective as of June 23, 20 ___, by and between Winter School District, of Winter, Wisconsin, herein referred to as *District* and Quality Therapy Resources, of Blue Lake, Wisconsin, herein referred to as *Agency*.

Description of Services. Beginning on August 23, 20 ___ and terminating on May 30, 20___, Agency will provide school occupational therapy services, including evaluation of children designated by the District director of special education; documentation of evaluation; participation in individualized education program (IEP) team meetings; development of treatment plans; provision of amount of occupational therapy intervention in IEPs; travel between schools; and communication and collaboration with school staff and parents. Agency will provide service in accordance with the standards of practice in state law.

Qualified Personnel. Agency will designate as the Service Provider a person who is licensed as an OT by the Wisconsin Department of Regulation and Licensing and licensed as a school OT by the Wisconsin Department of Public Instruction for the duration of the Agreement. Agency will provide district with copies of said licenses within four working days of the beginning of the service. Agency will provide replacement personnel with equal qualifications if the Service Provider is unable to provide services to District during the term of the Agreement. Agency will be responsible for professional liability coverage of Service Provider and replacement personnel.

Payment for Services. District will pay compensation to Agency for the services based on $_____ per hour. District will reimburse mileage at the rate of ____, based on monthly documentation of actual miles driven. Compensation shall be payable upon receipt of monthly billing statement from Agency. Service Provider will submit to District a monthly log of service activities. District will approve in advance any compensated activities other than those described in this agreement.

Termination. This Agreement may be terminated by either party upon 30 days written notice to the other party.

Confidentiality. Agency will protect and maintain the confidentiality of pupil records and patient health care records that District maintains, as required by state and federal law. This provision shall continue to be effective after the termination of this Agreement. Upon termination of this Agreement, Agency will return to District all records, documentation, and other items that were used, created, or controlled by Agency during the term of this Agreement.

Renewal. Renewal of this Agreement shall be based on District evaluation of quality of service and Agency availability to provide service.

Entire Agreement. This Agreement contains the entire agreement of the parties and there are no other promised or conditions in any other agreement whether oral or written.

Severability. If any provision of this Agreement shall be held to be invalid or unenforceable for any reason, the remaining provisions shall continue to be valid and enforceable.

Party purchasing services:
Winter School District
By: _____

     Jane Q. Superintendent
     District Administrator

Party providing services:
Quality Therapy Resources

By: _____

     Quality Therapy Resources
     President

Note: The district should review the purchase of service agreement with the district's legal counsel prior to entering into a contractual agreement.

Districts, therapists, and assistants should be aware that private agencies may have noncompete clauses in contracts. An example that might be included in a contract follows.

The district will not employ or solicit the employment of an agency therapist or assistant during the term of the agreement and for a period of one year after the termination of this agreement unless the agency gives its prior written consent. Such consent may be granted or withheld at the agency's sole discretion. To the extent the agency may agree to grant any such consent, a flat fee of $7,500 per therapist or assistant will be paid to the agency by the district prior to receipt of such written consent. In case of breach of this provision by the district, the district agrees to pay the agency, as liquidated damages and not as a penalty, the amount of $10,000 per therapist or assistant. This agreement in no way prohibits the agency or any of the agency's therapists or assistants from contracting with any other entity during or after the term hereof. (Dominiczak Therapy Associates 2009)

The Interview

The director or other administrator participates in an interview of prospective therapists. Whether the district hires a therapist through a school contract or purchase-of-service agreement, the director can gather information needed to make a hiring decision and determine staff development needs through portfolio review, team interview, and reference review.

Portfolio Review

In a portfolio review, the candidate or agency provides copies of reports for two or three children recently served. The children's full names should be redacted to maintain confidentiality. The therapist with school-based experience provides sample evaluations, IEPs, treatment plans, and progress notes. The director reviews these samples for clarity, with the following questions in mind.

- Is the educational impact of the disability clearly stated?

- Is a recommendation for or against therapy in school based on the child's needs in school?

- Is the IEP an integrated document, rather than one that contains pages specific to individual services?

- Is objective data collected to monitor progress?

- Do progress notes document actual services provided and the student's response to intervention?

The therapist without school experience provides reports on clients previously served. The director reviews these for statements of the functional impact of the client's disability, and the therapist's plans to increase functional activity.

Team Interview

Optimally, the interview team consists of the building principal or special education director and an OT or PT, with the possible addition of an IEP team coordinator or school psychologist, a teacher of special education, and a parent. If labor agreements prohibit involvement of certain staff in personnel decisions, those staff members may provide interview questions for the director or principal to use. When hiring a PT, the interview team could review "Updated Competencies for Physical Therapists Working in Schools" noted in chapter 5. The competencies provide the interview team with an overview of the knowledge and skills that a school-based PT should have or needs to acquire to provide quality care for students with disabilities at school. A candidate may not meet all of the nine competencies, but the team decides if the district could provide the opportunities and resources to enhance the professional knowledge and skills of the therapist for school-based practice.

The team decides if the district could provide the opportunities and resources to enhance the professional knowledge and skills of the therapist.

The team conducts the direct interview process for the therapist as they would for any long-term professional employee in the district. Interview issues that are specific to the position include IEP team and evaluation procedures, IEPs and rationale for services relevant to school, and team communication and collaboration skills.

Reference Review

The candidate provides professional references from three sources:

1. administrative or supervisory personnel, who can comment on the collaborative skills and technical skills of the therapist

2. professional peers, who can comment on the collaborative skills and technical skills of the therapist

3. direct service recipients, such as a parent, child, or special education teacher who can comment on the direct and indirect services provided by the therapist

Orientation

The director introduces the OT, PT, OTA, or PTA to principals, teachers, and parents in written correspondence. The director orients the newly hired therapist in person to local policy, procedures, and practices regarding occupational therapy or physical therapy in the educational setting, including scheduling, caseloads, workloads, equipment and space, documentation requirements, supervision, and evaluation of personnel and services.

The mentor assists the new therapist with working as a collaborative partner.

The director may assign a staff member to serve as a mentor during the first year the therapist is with the district. The mentor assists the new therapist with working as a collaborative partner on the IEP team, consulting with school staff, and meeting documentation procedures specific to the district. The director may contact the therapist at regular intervals during the first several months to determine if the therapist understands and is able to carry out district practices. Reference materials, including this guide, the Chapter PI 11, Wis. Admin Code regarding special education and related services, and the district policy and procedures manual for staff will assist the OT or PT in meeting the requirements of the position. At the beginning of the school year, WOTA provides an online orientation course for OTs, PTs, OTAs and PTAs new to school-based practice. The course provides an overview of special education law, assessment, IEPs, treatment plans, service delivery models, OTA and PTA supervision, differentiation of school-based and community-based services, paperwork, networking, and assistive technology. Directors can encourage new therapy personnel to attend this session as part of orientation. Conference information is found under continuing education on the WOTA website at http://www.wota.net/

The professional relationship of a therapist with a school district begins with an appropriate position description.

Assuring Quality

Quality assurance in school occupational and physical therapy is the joint responsibility of administrators and therapists. Therapists must have clear information from administrators about the expectations and policies of the school district and administrators and about their responsibilities under state and federal law. Administrators must have a working understanding from therapists of the roles and contributions of therapists to the educational process. The professional relationship of a therapist with a school district begins with an appropriate position description and an accurate assessment of the time a therapist will require to fulfill the expectations of the district. During the interview and orientation period, the director or other administrator and the therapist identify knowledge and skills in which the therapist is proficient, and knowledge and skills the therapist must develop to assure quality service in the school district. Together, they formulate and implement a professional development plan. They also develop a plan for managing and evaluating the effectiveness and efficiency of the specific related service as a whole, if one is not already in place. This collaboration forms a foundation for future evaluations of the quality of the related service.

Evaluating Staff Performance

School administrators can readily assess the performance of related service staff in the school setting by observing staff performing essential job activities, surveying those who work with related service staff, and reviewing records. The essential activities in the job performance of school therapists include

- participating in IEP team meetings.

- participating in IEP development.

- providing direct services, both individual and group.

- providing indirect services through collaboration with other staff.

- documenting services.

- communicating and collaborating with children, parents, teachers, other therapists and assistants, administrators, and physicians.

In addition to these activities, which are described in detail in other chapters of this guide, therapists assist in the management of their respective programs; educate other therapists and educators; supervise assistants and student therapists; and monitor and maintain their own professional growth and adherence to professional ethics.

The director, building principal, or other administrator follows performance appraisal criteria based on the therapist's position description when evaluating the performance of therapy staff, and the administrator, the therapist, or both may develop those criteria. APTA provides resources that may assist directors and therapists in evaluating PTs' performance. PTs may find these APTA publications helpful: *Clinical Skills Performance Evaluation Tools for Physical Therapists—Pediatrics, Assessing Competence: A Resource Manual* (APTA 2003[1]), and *Professionalism in Physical Therapy: Core Values Self Assessment.* (APTA 2003[2]) Both the PT and director could refer to the *Updated Competencies for Physical Therapists Working in Schools* noted in chapter 5 and develop a checklist to assess the therapist's performance and plan for the therapist's professional development. Figure 30 on pages 186 through 191 illustrates a sample form an administrator could use to document performance evaluation. OTs can assist administrators in evaluating best practices by self-appraisal of competency in the roles and responsibilities described in chapter 4, or by the use of a self-appraisal tool like *Developing, Maintaining and Updating Competency in Occupational Therapy: A Guide to Self Appraisal.* (Hinojosa et al. 1995) Many educational administrators find it difficult to evaluate the quality of treatment or intervention. The quality of intervention is reflected in

- the documented achievement of outcomes related to the child's IEP goals and objectives.

- the ability of therapists to articulate the link between the evaluations and intervention they provide to projected functional outcomes for the child in the school environment.

- the use of research-based practices to the extent practicable.

Administrators can assist therapists in developing school-related outcome measures that demonstrate improved ability of children to function in the child's current educational environment. Administrators and therapists may address specific questions about appropriate assessment and intervention by bringing in a consultant who has specific training in the therapy area and who is familiar with the objectives of school-based practice.

Single-case studies and qualitative research emerged as alternatives to control group studies.

Figure 30 Sample Performance Appraisals

Occupational Therapist

Rate each element of performance using the numerical values below. Average each heading (evaluation, planning, intervention, supervision, and other) to determine appraisal.

1 = unsatisfactory
2 = needs improvement
3 = meets expectations
4 = exceeds expectations
0 = not applicable

Evaluation

Reviews existing information following appointment to IEP team and prior to evaluating child. ___
Evaluates child using procedures to help determine eligibility and educational needs. ___
Documents in an individual report
     identifying and background information about child ___
     description of evaluation procedures ___
     summary and analysis of evaluation findings ___
     child's functional abilities and deficits in occupational performance areas
     and components ___
     projected functional outcomes for child as a result of intervention
     recommendations ___
Communicates and interprets results to the IEP team including parents ___
Complies with confidentiality and consent laws and standards. ___
Adheres to time frames required by law and school district policy. ___

Comments:
_____
_____

Planning

Collaborates with school personnel and parents to develop an IEP. ___
Recommends appropriate contexts and models for occupational therapy intervention ___
Identifies assistive technology necessary to implement the IEP. ___
Discusses community resources that may benefit the child. ___
Documents an occupational therapy treatment plan based on the IEP. ___

Comments:
_____
_____

Intervention

Obtains relevant medical information prior to providing intervention. ___
Implements the occupational therapy treatment plan. ___
Collaborates with other school personnel and parents to provide services. ___
Evaluates and documents the child's occupational performance areas and
components periodically. ___
Modifies intervention based on child's response and progress toward goals. ___
Provides the amount, frequency and duration of occupational therapy specified in
the IEP. ___
Discusses discontinuance of occupational therapy at IEP team meeting. ___
Documents comparison of initial status and status at time of discontinuance in terms
of occupational performance areas and components. ___
Documents recommendations for child following discontinuance of service.

Comments: _____

_____

Supervision

Determines and adheres to appropriate level of supervision for occupational ___
therapy assistants (OTAs).
Determines service competency of OTAs and delegates therapy for selected ___
children. ___
Documents supervisory visits and modifications of children's treatment plans. ___
Supervises student OTs and student OTAs.
Communicates expectations clearly and collaborates with OTA or student to solve ___
problems.
Comments:_____

_____

Other

Maintains licensure and continuing education as required by law. ___
Adheres to school district policies. ___
Maintains records required by Medicaid or insurance payers. ___
Maintains equipment, supplies, and designated space. ___
Evaluates the service and performs quality improvement activities. ___
Provides in-service education to other team members, parents, or community. ___
Monitors own performance and identifies supervisory and continuing education ___
needs.
Comments:

_____

_____

Evaluator's summary comments:_____

_____

Occupational therapist's summary comments: _____

_____

_____

_____   _____
Evaluator's Signature   Date Signed

_____   _____
Occupational Therapist Signature   Date Signed

Source: OT 4 and PI 11.24, Wisconsin Administrative Code; American Occupational Therapy
Association, (1993). Occupational therapy roles. American Journal of Occupational Therapy, 47,
1087-1090.; American Occupational Therapy Association, (1995). Elements of clinical
documentation (Revision). American Journal of Occupational Therapy, 49, 1032-1035.

Physical Therapist

Rate each element of performance using the numerical values below. Average each heading (evaluation, planning, intervention, supervision, and other) to determine appraisal.

1 = unsatisfactory
2 = needs improvement
3 = meets expectations
4 = exceeds expectations
0 = not applicable

Evaluation

Reviews existing data and seeks medical information prior to providing physical therapy service. ___
Evaluates child using appropriate physical therapy pediatric assessment tools. ___
Identifies child's ability to participate in school activities. ___
Identifies child's ability to move throughout the school environment. ___
Communicates and interprets results to the IEP team. ___
Complies with confidentiality and consent laws and standards. ___

Comments:

_____

Planning

Collaborates with IEP team to develop child's IEP. ___
Recommends appropriate physical therapy services. ___
Identifies assistive technology necessary to implement the IEP. ___
Documents a physical therapy treatment plan based on the IEP. ___
___

Comments:

_____

Intervention

Implements the physical therapy treatment plan, ___
Modifies treatment plan based on child's response and progress toward goals. ___
Collaborates with other school personnel and parents to provide services. ___
Records treatment provided, child's progress, and change in child's status on an ongoing basis. ___
Provides the amount, frequency, and duration of physical therapy specified in the IEP. ___

Comments:

_____

Supervision

Determines appropriate level of supervision for physical therapist assistants (PTAs). ___
Determines service competency of PTAs and delegates therapy for selected children. ___
Documents supervisory visits and modifications of children's treatment plans. ___
Supervises student PTs and student PTAs.

Comments:

_____

Other

Maintains licensure as required by law. ___

Adheres to school district policies. ___

Maintains records required by Medicaid or insurance payers. ___

Maintains equipment, supplies, and designated space. ___

Evaluates the service and performs quality improvement activities. ___

Provides in-service education to other team members, parents, or community. ___

Monitors own performance and identifies supervisory and continuing education needs. ___

Comments:

_____

Evaluator's summary
comments:_____

_____

Physical therapist's summary
comments_____

_____

_____   _____
Evaluator's Signature   Date Signed

_____   _____
Physical Therapist Signature   Date Signed

Source: American Physical Therapy Association (January 1996). Standards of practice for physical therapy. PT Magazine of Physical Therapy; P 11.24, Wisconsin Administrative Code.

Occupational Therapy Assistant

Rate each element of performance using the numerical values below. Average each heading (evaluation, planning, intervention, supervision, and other) to determine appraisal.

    1 = unsatisfactory
    2 = needs improvement
    3 = meets expectations
    4 = exceeds expectations
    0 = not applicable

Evaluation

Assists the occupational therapist (OT) with data collection and evaluation. ____
Assists the OT with recording and documenting evaluation results. ____
Complies with confidentiality and consent laws and standards. ____

Comments:

_____

Planning

Assists the OT in developing an occupational therapy treatment plan. ____
Establishes service competence in collaboration with the OT for designated intervention procedures. ____

Comments:

_____

Intervention

Implements the occupational therapy treatment plan under the supervision of the OT. ____
Collaborates with other school personnel and parents to provide services. ____
Documents intervention procedures and the child's response. ____
Recommends modifications of intervention to the OT. ____
Adapts environments, tools, materials, and activities as the child needs. ____
Comments: _____

Other

Maintains licensure and continuing education as required by law. ____
Adheres to school district policies. ____
Maintains equipment, supplies, and designated space. ____
Assists the OT in: ____
    maintaining recordkeeping and reporting system. ____
    evaluating the service and performing quality improvement activities. ____
    providing inservice education to other team members, parents, or community. ____
    providing fieldwork experience to OT and OTA students. ____
Monitors own performance and identifies supervisory and continuing education needs. ____
Comments: _____

Evaluator's summary comments:

_____
_____

Occupational therapy assistant's summary comments:

_____
_____

_____   _____
Evaluator's Signature   Date Signed

_____   _____
Occupational Therapist Assistant Signature   Date Signed

Physical Therapist Assistant

Rate each element of performance using the numerical values below. Average each heading (evaluation, planning, intervention, supervision, and other) to determine appraisal.

    1 = unsatisfactory
    2 = needs improvement
    3 = meets expectations
    4 = exceeds expectations
    0 = not applicable

Evaluation

Assists the physical therapist with data collection.   ____
Assists the physical therapist with recording and documenting evaluation results.   ____
Complies with confidentiality and consent laws and standards.   ____

Comments:

_____

Planning

Establishes service competence in collaboration with the physical therapist for designated intervention procedures.   ____

Comments:

_____

Intervention

Implements the physical therapy treatment plan under the supervision of the physical therapist.   ____
Collaborates with other school personnel and parents to provide services.   ____
Documents intervention procedures and the child's response.   ____
Makes modifications in interventions as directed by the physical therapist or to ensure student's safety.   ____
Adapts environments, tools, materials, and activities as the child needs.   ____

Comments:

_____

Other

Maintains licensure as required by law.   ____
Adheres to school district policies.   ____
Maintains equipment, supplies, and designated space.   ____
Assists the physical therapist in: ____
    maintaining recordkeeping and reporting system.   ____
    evaluating the service and performing quality improvement activities.   ____
    providing in-service education to other team members, parents, or community.   ____
Monitors own performance and identifies supervisory and education needs.   ____

Comments:

_____

Evaluator's summary comments:_____

_____

Physical therapist assistant's summary comments: _____

_____

_____   _____
Evaluator's Signature   Date Signed

_____   _____
Occupational Therapist Assistant Signature   Date Signed

District Contracted Staff

Therapists who are hired under a district's master agreement undergo evaluation in accordance with that agreement. This process may include a review of recent IEPs, professional documentation, and an interview or a survey of those working directly with the therapist. The evaluation process is finalized when the therapist and administrator create and implement a professional development plan.

Purchase-of-Service Staff

The administrator annually assesses the ability of purchase-of-service staff to meet the service expectations of the district prior to contract renewal. Although many districts contract annually for purchase-of-service staff, there will be times when the contract will run for a shorter amount of time. In this case, administrators should plan for an exit interview, or quarterly meetings with the contracted agency. The administrator may collaborate with the contracting agency during the assessment of staff performance. The purchase-of-service agreement should specify the expectation of ongoing assessment of performance and need for professional development.

Evaluating Outcomes

In recent years, people across the nation have become interested in the cost and outcomes of both special education and health care. Studies in both fields have measured outcomes of techniques that educators and therapists use. Single-case studies and qualitative research emerged as alternatives to control group studies, which were sometimes of questionable value considering the wide diversity among children in any single category of disability, and the effects of the relationship between the child and the educator or therapist. Within a school district of Cooperative Educational Service Agency (CESA), OTs, PTs, and administrators evaluate the outcomes of therapy provided to each child, as well as the overall impact of occupational therapy and physical therapy services on the child's education. In order to measure individual outcomes with children, therapists must conduct evaluations that are relevant to the child's function in school; establish baseline data against which the therapist and educator can measure progress; and document the child's activities in relation to goals, at regular intervals. In order to measure overall service outcomes, the therapist and director must collaborate with others to examine the outcome data from all children, as well as the collective performance of therapists and assistants in relation to the school district's expectations. In a complex, dynamic system like school, conflicting expectations may exist. An honest appraisal of service outcome requires the participants to identify the expectations of the therapists, teachers, principals, directors of special education, parents, school district administrators, and school board members in order to know what standard is the standard of quality.

A tool that districts can use to measure the effectiveness of school-based therapy is the School Outcomes Measure (SOM). SOM was developed by the University of Oklahoma Health Sciences Center, Department of Rehabilitation

In a complex, dynamic system like school, conflicting expectations may exist.

Science, 2007. The SOM is a minimal data set designed to collect data from students with disabilities who receive school-based occupational therapy, physical therapy, or both. A minimal data set is a standardized outcome measure that includes the fewest number of items possible to provide the information needed. It is designed to collect population-based data across individuals to identify outcomes for people with particular characteristics and interventions.

Equipment

Specialized equipment is often necessary for the implementation of occupational therapy and physical therapy. A student may need this equipment to gain access to or participate in an activity, or to participate in educational activities that the therapist develops. Having appropriate equipment is integral to conducting interventions designed to increase the participation of the student in school activities. When considering procurement of equipment, school staff and administrators consider whether the equipment is necessary to allow students to benefit from special education, either directly or through the continued use of the equipment in the classroom or other school setting. *Equipment* can be categorized as

- items essential for health or safety in school activities, such as aerosol disinfectant, floor mats, toilet support systems, and seating systems.

- evaluation tools, such as test kits, forms, or videotapes.

- basic equipment used with a variety of children over a period of years, such as stacking benches, adapted utensils, a therapy ball, or a stopwatch.

- supplies used with a variety of children for the duration of a school term, such as multiple sizes of crayons and markers, small toys and other items to reinforce behavior or manipulate during learning activities.

Some districts include occupational therapy and physical therapy equipment, test kits, and other materials on the IDEA flow-through budget. More information about equipment is in chapter 7 and Appendix E.

Facilities

Occupational therapy and physical therapy often require designated space in the general education environment or special education setting where they are often integrated. Designated space is necessary when the activities of assessment or therapy are disruptive to the classroom; when the student needs specific stationary equipment; or when the student needs a private area with minimal distraction. Areas of designated space for students should be clean, well-lit, and well-ventilated. There should be a telephone or intercom system in the event of an emergency and should have facilities for therapists to wash their hands.

Staff needs for designated space include access to a private telephone for calls to physicians, parents, and private agencies; a locked storage area for equipment, files, and materials; and an area for record keeping and report writing. *Space and Facilities* in chapter 2 provides more information.

Changes in Staff

A school district should anticipate that staff resignations or leaves will occur. The director notifies parents, principals, and staff indicating the nature of the change, the effective date of change, resulting schedule changes, and activities that will occur during the transition. The director facilitates a smooth transition by ensuring that the departing therapist has materials and information in place and organized for the new therapist. This includes IEPs; treatment plans; attendance records; progress notes; and other documentation, such as names of other school staff and personnel outside of the district who serve a child. The departing therapist should identify where the new therapist can locate equipment, supplies, assessment tools, keys, computers, and available office facilities in various buildings.

The director facilitates a smooth transition by ensuring that the departing therapist has materials and information in place and organized for the new therapist.

Reimbursement

Wisconsin school districts and CESAs fund the provision of occupational therapy and physical therapy through local revenues, state aids, and federal funds. State and federal funding sources include Wisconsin Medical Assistance Program, or Medicaid; State Handicapped Child Categorical Aid; and IDEA Flow-through and Preschool funds.

Medicaid

Wisconsin Act 27 of 1995 established the Medicaid School Based Services benefit (SBS). The benefit allows schools to bill Wisconsin Medicaid for medically necessary services that schools provide to Medicaid-eligible children, if the school district obtains informed parental consent. (Wisconsin Department of Public Instruction 2007 and 2009) The services may include occupational therapy or physical therapy.

A school district or CESA can become a Medicaid provider by applying for certification from Medicaid's fiscal agent. Individual school therapists do not become certified providers under the SBS benefit, but they must be DPI-licensed therapists before Medicaid will reimburse a school district or CESA for their services. Medicaid defines an SBS as medically necessary when the service

A school district or CESA can become a Medicaid provider by applying for certification from Medicaid's fiscal agent.

- identifies, treats, manages, or addresses a medical problem, or a mental, emotional or physical disability.

- is identified in an IEP or Individualized Family Service Program (IFSP).

- allows a child to benefit from special education.

- is prescribed by a physician when required.

Covered services for both occupational therapy and physical therapy include

- evaluation and re-evaluation to determine the child's need for these services and recommendations for a course of treatment.

- individual therapy or treatment or group therapy or treatment in groups of 2-7 children.

- medical equipment identified in the IEP intended for only one child for use at school and home.

The physician's prescription requirements for occupational therapy and physical therapy are waived if the district has a *Request of a Waiver to Wisconsin Medicaid Prescription Requirements under the SBS* on file with Medicaid. Districts can find the waiver form on the DHS website at http://dhs.wisconsin.gov/forms/F0/F01134.pdf. Districts may also submit a waiver for close supervision of OTAs and PTAs. Districts can find the waiver form, Wisconsin Medicaid Request for Waiver of Physical Therapist Assistant and Occupational Therapy Assistant Supervision Requirement on the DHS website at http://dhs.wisconsin.gov/forms/F0/F01149.doc. School therapists should remember that SBS requires the supervising therapist to co-sign the assistant's entry in a medical record.

Flow-through and Preschool Budgets

IDEA flow-through and preschool entitlement budgets are part of the Local Performance Plan districts submit to DPI. Districts may use these federal funds for therapists' salaries and fringe benefits, purchased services such as contracted therapy, and items such as test kits or therapy equipment. Salaries and fringe benefits paid with federal funds are not eligible for state handicapped child categorical aid.

State Handicapped Child Categorical Aid

School districts must follow requirements and reporting procedures to obtain state categorical reimbursement for part of the salaries and fringe benefits of school OTs, PTs, OTAs, and PTAs.

The school district or CESA that is the hiring agency reports their names, social security numbers, FTEs, salary, fringe, years of experience, highest degree earned, grades served, or whether services are privately contracted on the third Friday in September. The district or CESA submits this information on the web-based application on the PI 1202 Fall Staff Report. The director must ensure that each therapist and assistant, including those provided by a contract agency, has a current and appropriate DPI license. The Department verifies licenses and reimburses districts and CESAs based on license status.

The director must ensure that each therapist and assistant, including those provided by a contract agency, has a current and appropriate DPI license.

Records

In Wisconsin, students' education records are called pupil records, and they refer to all records directly related to a student and maintained by the school district. Pupil records include records maintained in any way including, but not limited to, computer storage media, video and audio tape, film, microfilm, and microfiche. There are three basic kinds of pupil records: behavioral records, progress records, and patient health care records, and the definitions that follow are all from Wisconsin Statutes.

Behavioral Records

Behavioral records means those pupil records which include psychological tests; personality evaluations; records of conversations; any written statement relating specifically to an individual pupil's behavior; tests relating specifically to achievement or measurement of ability; the pupil's physical health records other than immunization records or lead screening records required under s. 254.162, Wis. Stats.; law enforcement officers' records obtained under s. 48.396(1) or s. 938.396(1m), Wis. Stats.; and any other pupil records that are not progress records. s.118.125(1)(a),Wis. Stats.

Progress Records

Progress records means those pupil records which include the pupil's grades, a statement of the courses the pupil has taken, the pupil's attendance record, the pupil's immunization records, any lead screening records required under s. 254.162, Wis. Stats., and the records of the pupil's extracurricular activities. s.118.125(1)(c), Wis. Stats.

Patient Health Care Records

Patient health care records within a school are any pupil record that relates to a pupil's health and that do not fall within the definition of pupil physical health record. s.118.125(2m), Wis. Stats. In general, records relating to the health of a child that contain such information as diagnoses, opinions, and judgments made by a health care provider, except for records containing only the basic health information included in the definition of pupil physical health records, are treated as patient health care records.

Wisconsin law classifies the documents school OTs and PTs write as *pupil records*. The pupil records that school OTs and PTs prepare, alone or in collaboration with others, are usually either behavioral records or patient health care records. *Patient health care records* are all records related to the health of a patient, prepared by or under the supervision of a health care provider. The definition of *health care provider* includes OTs, PTs, OTAs, and PTAs. (s.146.81, Wis. Stats.)

Privacy and Security

The Family Educational Rights and Privacy Act (FERPA) is the Federal law that protects the privacy of students' education records. In 1996, Congress enacted the Health Insurance Portability and Accountability Act (HIPAA) to protect the privacy and security of individually identifiable health information. When schools maintain patient health care records, the state considers the information pupil records, and thus subject to FERPA rules, not HIPAA. However, when a school wants or needs health information from outside health care providers, schools need to adhere to the disclosure requirement of the outside health care providers (which are HIPAA-governed) to gain access to the information. As part of an IEP evaluation, the district may want to review existing data in a student's patient health care record from a clinic or hospital. This requires a signed release form from the parent. The form should include the names of all IEP team members that require access to the reports and records. In the event of a student transferring to another school district, patient health care records that originated outside of the original district should not be forwarded to the new district. Patient health care records generated in the school district can be forwarded to another school district. This includes the school-based therapists' reports.

When schools maintain patient health care records, the state considers the information pupil records, and thus subject to FERPA rules, not HIPAA.

Districts may adopt a policy that only educationally relevant information will be included in reports. The reports are then considered behavioral records, not patient health care records. However, PTs' reports typically contain information and professional terminology related to current health status, health history, functional status and activity level, tests and measures, types of interventions, and clinical judgment about response to intervention and expected outcomes. This information reflects patient health care data and the document would be filed as a patient health care record. S. 448.56(5), Wis. Stats. requires a PT to create and maintain a patient record and this more closely aligns with a patient health care record. PTs may be able to write some reports, such as progress reports using only educationally relevant information and this documentation would be considered a behavior record and stored accordingly.

The standards of practice, Chapter OT 4, Wis. Admin Code, requires OTs to document the evaluation including the specific evaluation tools and methods; the intervention plan including the student's occupational performance areas, occupational performance components and occupational performance contexts; and the discontinuation of services with a comparison of the initial and current state of functional abilities and deficits in occupational performance areas and occupational performance components. This documentation typically contains professional terminology and medical information, so it would be filed and stored as patient health care information. OTs may be able to write other reports, such as progress reports, using only educationally relevant information and this documentation would then be considered a behavior record and stored accordingly.

Disclosure

A school district may disclose personally identifiable information from a pupil record under three circumstances: signed release form from parent, guardian or adult student; court order; or by authority of statute. Legally, pupil records must be made available to district employed DPI certified staff and other school officials that the school board determines to have legitimate educational interests, including safety interests s.118.125(2)(d), Wis. Stats. School boards designate contracted therapists as school district officials with an educational interest in pupil records. Patient health care records may be released without informed consent to school district employees if access is necessary to comply with a requirement in federal or state law, such as IDEA or Chapter PI 11, Wis. Admin Code. Districts may limit independent access to patient health care records to only those staff who are qualified to interpret the information. The law also grants access to patient health care records to persons who prepare or store the records, such as school office staff. Districts document all disclosures including what was disclosed, to whom records were disclosed, date of disclosure, and authorization for the disclosure.

Patient health care records may be released without informed consent if access is necessary to comply with a requirement in federal or state law.

Maintenance

The department recommends patient health care records be maintained separately from other pupil records because the requirements relating to access to and disclosure of information from patient health care records are more restrictive than the requirements for other pupil records. If a district stores patient health care records in the same file as behavioral records, or therapists include patient or family health care information in evaluation reports, they may inadvertently violate the confidentiality of the child's patient health care records by making them available to all school staff. Notes or personal records of a school therapist which are not shown or shared with others are not pupil records s.115.28(7), Wis. Stats. If a therapist shares part or all of the contents of the note or personal record, the information becomes a pupil record and must be treated as such.

Categorizing information specifically as a pupil record also determines how long the school must retain the record. The school must keep progress records for at least five years after the pupil is no longer enrolled. The school may keep behavioral records no more than one year after the pupil is no longer enrolled, unless the pupil consents in writing to an extended period of record retention. No existing statutory language governs retention of patient health care records in schools.

The school board adopts and publishes its policy on record retention, and should include a statement on retaining patient health care records. The Wisconsin Medical Assistance Program advises schools that bill Medicaid to retain records related to claims for five years. In addition to board policy, contracts between the school and a health care provider, such as an OT or PT, should address where and how long the provider will keep patient health care records of students served.

More information is available in *Student Records and Confidentiality* on the department's website at http://dpi.wi.gov/sspw/pdf/srconfid.pdf. Information about access to records is found at http://dpi.wi.gov/sped/accessrecords.html.

Electronic Mail (E-Mail)

Therapists need to be aware of and adhere to school district policies regarding e-mail use. E-mail messages are public records and are subject to open records law, investigatory review, or discovery proceedings in legal actions. Therapists should use professional judgment when communicating electronically and consider the message a professional document. This is important to remember as e-mail tends to be regarded generally as an informal and casual conversation between private individuals. Therapists and other school staff should not communicate via e-mail about specific students as this is a violation of student confidentiality.

Liability

"Risk management is the process of identifying, analyzing, and addressing areas of existing and potential risk." (APTA 2009) School therapists apply risk *management practices to provide students with interventions, activities, and* adaptive equipment in an environment which poses low risk. Districts may have a risk management/safety team and a school-based therapist may be a member of the team. Therapists need to comply with district safety and risk management policies and procedures. The professional organizations, AOTA and APTA, provide guidance on risk management on their respective websites and in publications and other documents.

"Proactive risk management practices can help avoid or reduce liability." (APTA 2009) Most school districts provide liability insurance for their employees, but all therapists, whether they are hired by the district, working independently, or hired by a CESA or other agency, should consider carrying their own insurance. It is the responsibility of school OTs and PTs to have adequate liability insurance against claims of negligence or malpractice.

Therapists should consider carrying their own insurance.

A hearing or court proceeding may require a therapist to submit documentation of a student's services as evidence. As therapists write reports and keep records, they should keep in mind that courts or hearing officers could use these records to support or refute a litigant's allegations. To protect themselves and the students they serve, therapists should follow professional practice documentation guidelines. Documentation of proper use of equipment, regular maintenance of equipment and sufficient training of other staff have been factors in the resolution of complaints to DPI, as described in chapter 7.

References

American Occupational Therapy Association. 2006. "Transforming *Caseload* to *Workload* in School-Based and Early Intervention Occupational Therapy Services." Bethesda, MD: American Occupational Therapy Association. http://www.aota.org/Practitioners/PracticeAreas/Pediatrics/Browse/School/38519.aspx (accessed August 18, 2010).

American Physical Therapy Association. 2003[1]. *Clinical Skills Performance Evaluation Tools for Physical Therapists – Pediatrics.* Alexandria, VA: American Physical Therapy Association.

___."Professionalism in Physical Therapy: Core Values Self-Assessment." 2003[2]. http://www.apta.org/AM/Template.cfm?Section=Professionalism1&TEMPLATE=/CM/ContentDisplay.cfm&CONTENTID=41460 (accessed August 18, 2010).

___. "Physical Therapy Workforce Project: Physical Therapy Vacancy and Turnover Rates in Acute Care Hospitals, February 28, 2008," http://www.apta.org/AM/Template.cfm?Section=Demographics&CONTENTID=46601&TEMPLATE=/CM/ContentDisplay.cfm (accessed March 9, 2010 - members only).

___. "Risk Management." 2009. http://www.apta.org/AM/PrinterTemplate.cfm?Section=Risk_Management2&Template=/TaggedPage/TaggedPageDisplay.cfm&TPLID=312&ContentID=37579 (accessed August 18, 2010).

Cecere, S. 2008. "School-based Special Interest Group, Workload Subcommittee Report." *APTA's Section on Pediatrics School-Based Special Interest Group (SIG) Newsletter* 4-6.

___. 2010. "School SIG's Workload Study: Descriptive Statistics." *APTA's Section on Pediatrics, School-Based PT Special Interest Group Newsletter* 5.

Center on Personnel Studies in Special Education (COPSSE) website. "Special Education Work Force Watch, Insights from Research." http://www.copsse.org/ (accessed February 2004).

Chiang, B., and B. Rylance. 2000. "Occupational and Physical Therapy Caseload Size: Service Provision and Perceptions of Efficacy." *Wisconsin Educators' Caseload Efficacy Project, Research Report 5.* University of Wisconsin–Oshkosh.

Hinojosa, J., L. Thomson, D. Lieberman, R. Murphy, E. Wendt, J. Poole, and S. Hertfelder. 1995. *Developing, Maintaining, and Updating Competency in Occupational Therapy: A Guide to Self-Appraisal.* Bethesda, MD: American Occupational Therapy Association.

University of Oklahoma Health Sciences Center, Department of Rehabilitation Science. "School Outcomes Measure, Administrative Guide 2007." http://www.ah.ouhsc.edu/somresearch/adminGuide.pdf (accessed March 9, 2010).

Wisconsin Department of Public Instruction. 2006. "Wisconsin Educator Supply and Demand Project" http://dpi.wi.gov/tepdl/pdf/supdem06.pdf (accessed March 18, 2010).

___. "Parent Consent to Bill Wisconsin Medicaid for Medically-related Special Education and/or Related Services." 2007. http://dpi.wi.gov/sped/bul07-02.html (accessed November 1, 2010).

___. "Student Records and Confidentiality." 2008. http://dpi.wi.gov/sspw/pdf/srconfid.pdf (accessed August 18, 2010).

___. "School-based Services (SBS) and Medicaid Administrative Claiming (MAC) – Student Confidentiality and Parental Consent." 2009. http://dpi.wi.gov/sped/bul09-01.html (accessed November 1, 2010).

Wisconsin Education Career Access Network (WECAN). http://services.education.wisc.edu/wecan (accessed August 18, 2010).

Wisconsin educator jobs and other jobs in educational settings. http://ww2.wisconsin.gov/state/employment/app?COMMAND=gov.wi.state.cpp. job.command.LoadSeekerHome (accessed August 18, 2010).

Wisconsin Occupational Therapy Association newsletter http://www.wota.net

Wisconsin Physical Therapy Association newsletter http://www.wpta.org/

Other Resources

American Physical Therapy Association. "School-based Special Interest Group News." 2008. http://www.pediatricapta.org/special-interest-groups/school-based-therapy/pdfs/School-Based%20SIG%20News%20-%20February%202008.pdf (accessed August 18, 2010).

Effgen, S., L. Chiarello, and S. Milbourne. 2007. "Updated Competencies for Physical Therapists Working in Schools." *Pediatric Physical Therapy* 19: 266-74.

"Joint Guidance on the Application of the *Family Educational Rights and Privacy Act (FERPA)* and the *Health Insurance Portability and Accountability Act of 1996 (HIPAA)* To Student Health Records." 2008. U.S. Department of Health and Humana Services and U.S. Department of Education.

Phillips, A. M. 2004. A*ssessing Competence: A Resource Manual.* Alexandria, VA: American Physical Therapy Association.

Questions and Answers

9

IEP Team

1. *How can teachers and other school staff recognize that a child may need occupational therapy or physical therapy as part of an Individualized Education Program (IEP)?*

   Teachers should identify the tasks and environments in which the child is not progressing or participating, try the educational accommodations or interventions that they think will support the child and monitor the child's response. The Reference Guides, Figures 6 and 7, in chapter 3 will help the teacher focus on areas that occupational therapy and physical therapy typically support.

2. *Does an occupational therapist need a medical referral?*

   No, provided the evaluation or intervention follows the IEP team process or the Section 504 process, and the occupational therapist (OT) or occupational therapy assistant (OTA) provides services in an educational environment, including the child's home, for a child with a disability. An OT requires medical information about a child with a disability before providing services. A physician's referral may be required if the OT serves a child who does not have a disability.

3. *Does a physical therapist need a medical referral?*

   No, with exception. A medical referral is not required when evaluating or serving a child with a disability under IDEA. A referral is also not required for other students when services are related to educational environments for conditioning, injury prevention, application of biomechanics, and treatment of musculoskeletal injuries. For provision of other services, a referral is needed. A medical referral is required when a student has an acute fracture, or soft tissue avulsion. A physical therapist (PT) requires medical information about a child with a disability from a physician before providing services.

4. *When must a school district include an occupational therapy or physical therapy evaluation as part of an IEP team process?*

   If the district suspects that a child needs occupational therapy or physical therapy, it must conduct an IEP team evaluation or reevaluation and hold a meeting to determine initially if the child requires occupational therapy or physical therapy. The district must conduct an IEP team reevaluation of a child at least every three years unless the district and the parent agree not to do so, and the reevaluation may include occupational therapy or physical therapy. If the child currently receives therapy and needs an assessment for another area of that therapy, such as assistive technology, the therapist may conduct the assessment without an IEP team process.

5. *May an OT legitimately screen a child for the need for occupational therapy? May a PT legitimately screen a child for the need for physical therapy?*

    No. Screening an individual child for the need for therapy is a form of evaluation, which includes observation, interview, and record review. The school district must have prior written notice and consent for evaluation from the parents for such an evaluation. The IEP team alone can determine if a child requires occupational therapy or physical therapy, following an evaluation by the respective therapist.

6. *How often must a therapist conduct an evaluation of a child?*

    The respective therapist must conduct an evaluation of the child when first assigned to the IEP team of a child suspected of needing occupational therapy or physical therapy. When a PT provides general supervision of a physical therapist assistant (PTA), the PT must provide an on-site reevaluation of each child's therapy a minimum of one time per calendar month or every tenth day of therapy, whichever is sooner. When an OT provides general supervision of an OTA, the OT must provide an on-site reevaluation of each child's therapy a minimum of one time per calendar month or every tenth day of therapy, whichever is sooner. The OT routinely evaluates and documents occupational performance areas and occupational performance components. As part of any IEP team reevaluation of a child who is receiving therapy, the IEP team reviews existing evaluation data and identifies whether any assessments or other evaluation measures must be administered to produce needed data.

7. *What process must an IEP team use to add occupational therapy or physical therapy to a child's existing IEP?*

    The school will conduct a reevaluation of a child, providing prior written notice to the parent and obtaining informed parental consent for evaluation as procedural safeguards, in order to consider adding occupational therapy or physical therapy to the IEP.

8. *Must the OT and the PT write individual reports of their evaluations as members of the IEP team?*

    Yes. The state license issued by the Wisconsin Department of Regulation and Licensing (DRL) to OTs requires that occupational therapy evaluation results be documented in the individual's record. The state license issued by DRL to PTs requires that PTs create a patient record for every patient the PT treats.

9. *Can the therapist recommend occupational therapy or physical therapy in the individual report?*

    Yes. The therapist may include in his or her report a statement concerning the nature of the therapy he or she recommends.

10. *What is the eligibility criterion for a child to receive occupational therapy or physical therapy?*

    The respective therapy must be required to assist the child to benefit from special education.

11. *Can a district use the following criterion: if the child's gross or fine motor level is commensurate with cognitive ability, then there is no need for therapy?*

    No. The fact that the child's delay in motor skill development is commensurate with the child's developmental levels in other areas is not an appropriate standard by which to determine a child's need for occupational therapy or physical therapy.

12. *Does the therapist decide if the child needs therapy?*

    The therapist makes a recommendation, but the IEP team determines if occupational therapy or physical therapy is required to assist the child to benefit from special education. This individualized decision is made most effectively after the team has written annual goals for the child and determined the special education that will help the child meet the goals. No other criterion, such as a test score, may be used as a qualification standard across all children.

13. *Can the OTA or PTA represent the therapist at the IEP team meeting?*

    No. The OTA or PTA cannot represent the therapist at the IEP team meeting. This would place the assistant in the position of interpreting findings and analyzing the student's need for therapy which is beyond the assistant's role and function. (PI 11.24(7)(e), Wis. Admin Code) The assistant may be able to provide therapy to the children while the therapist attends meetings.

IEP

1. *Should the OT and PT have their own pages on the IEP?*

    No. In the past, many educators and therapists brought different lists of instructional and therapy goals and objectives to the IEP meeting, often stapling these pages together to form the IEP. The team members should combine their efforts to develop the IEP *at the meeting.* The goals and objectives they set are for the child, not for the service providers. The child's occupational therapy and physical therapy treatment plans are the appropriate places to delineate the specific therapy goals and objectives.

2. *How do therapists and educators write functional goals and objectives?*
    Functional goals and objectives are written descriptions of what the child needs to do but is presently unable to do in a naturally occurring school environment. The IEP team writes goals and objectives that are the expected outcomes within those environments.

3. *Should IEP goals be general or specific?*
    The IEP team should write an annual goal with enough measurable indicators that anyone working with the child could determine if the child achieved the goal in a year. Goals and objectives are too specific if they begin to resemble treatment plans or daily instructional plans.

4. *How must occupational therapy and physical therapy be documented on the IEP?*
    Occupational therapy and physical therapy are related services. It is sufficient to check the box next to the service on the IEP (DPI form I-9) and to fill in amount, frequency, location and duration. Amount and frequency must be specific, either numbers, circumstances or both. Location should inform the IEP team of any time that the child is not with nondisabled peers. If the duration is a period of time different than the IEP duration, the beginning and ending date must be provided. The information should be clear to the IEP team and other teachers.

5. *How should the IEP team write the amount and frequency of therapy for infrequent consultation or for service that will vary in amount and frequency because of the child's needs?*
    In the case where it is impossible to describe special education services in daily or weekly allotments of time, the IEP must clearly describe the circumstances under which the service will be provided and for how long. This requires much more detail in the description of the therapy, such as *45 minutes total during the first week of each new unit in physical education.* Alternatively, the team may write a schedule into the IEP if they expect therapy to change in amount and frequency because of the child's future needs. This requires the team to predict the amount and frequency a child needs on specific dates.

6. *How does the amount and frequency of therapy on the IEPs relate to the amount of time a therapist is employed, the amount of time for which the school is billed, and the therapist's schedule?*
    The amount and frequency of therapy on the IEPs is one of several factors districts consider when determining the amount of time to employ or contract for a therapist. The therapist's schedule includes time to do the following: conduct evaluations; attend IEP team meetings and staff meetings; travel among buildings; set up and remove equipment and supplies; write reports, treatment plans and progress notes; contact parents

and physicians; and order equipment. An agency or CESA may bill a school district for an amount of time based on IEPs, but fees may be adjusted to account for the actual time the school requires from the therapist.

7. *May therapists cancel therapy to attend IEP team meetings or in-services?*
    No. Therapists may not cancel children's therapy to attend meetings if cancellation means the child will not receive the amount, frequency, and duration of therapy stated in the child's IEP. A school district either must hold an IEP meeting to change the amount, frequency, or duration of a child's therapy or must obtain the agreement of the child's parent to change the IEP without a meeting. However, when there is no change in the overall amount of therapy, the district may make some adjustments in scheduling without holding another IEP meeting.

8. *Must a therapist be excused in advance if he or she is unable to attend an IEP team meeting?*
    Yes. A school district may excuse a required member of an IEP team from attending a meeting in whole or in part if the child's parent agrees in writing. State law requires OTs, PTs, and speech pathologists to be IEP team members when a child needs or is suspected to need their respective services. When the meeting involves a modification to, or discussion of the therapist's service or area of the curriculum, any therapist who is excused from attending must give the parent and the IEP team written input into the development of the IEP prior to the meeting.

9. *Can the OT or PT recommend the amount and frequency of therapy if he or she is unable to attend the IEP team meeting?*
    Yes. The therapist may make a written recommendation concerning the nature, frequency, and amount of therapy to be provided to the child. The IEP team may consider the therapist's recommendation when they determine the content of the IEP.

10. *If the IEP team determines that specially-designed physical education is the only special education a child with an orthopedic impairment or other health impairment needs, can the child receive occupational therapy and physical therapy?*
    Yes. If the IEP team members determine the child requires occupational therapy and physical therapy to benefit from specially-designed physical education, then the child receives the related services.

11. *If a child is identified as having a speech and language impairment and also has sensory motor problems that significantly affect socialization at recess and manual activities in class, can the child receive occupational therapy?*
    Yes. Regardless of the child's area of impairment, the IEP team writes goals and objectives that address the unique academic and functional needs of the

child. It is up to each child's IEP team to determine the special education and related services needed to meet each child's unique needs in order for the child to receive a free, appropriate public education.

12. *If the therapist and other school staff in the IEP team meeting feel that discontinuing occupational therapy or physical therapy is appropriate but the parents disagree, who makes the final decision?*

School staff must consider parents' recommendations because they are equal participants in the IEP team meeting. It is helpful for the IEP team to identify the child's goals and the special education that will address the goals before asking if occupational therapy or physical therapy is required to assist the child to benefit from the special education that will be provided. IEP teams that cannot come to consensus may agree to pursue mediation or other methods of conflict resolution.

Caseload

1. *If a therapist's caseload exceeds the legal maximum, whose responsibility is it to reduce the number of children served by that therapist?*

The law permits caseloads to vary from the maximum numbers in law depending on factors that the law specifies. The amount of service in children's IEPs is one of those factors. The school district has a responsibility to provide the amount of service the IEP team has written into the IEP. Therapists and parents should bring caseload concerns to the attention of the school district's director of special education. Together, they should discuss management of the caseload, which may include reducing the therapist's caseload, adding staff, or allocating the therapist's time differently.

2. *Does the number of children on a therapist's caseload include children who receive infrequent consultation (periodic check)?*

Yes. When he or she receives direct or indirect therapy pursuant to an IEP, the child is counted on the therapist's caseload regardless of the frequency of therapy.

Documentation

1. *What type of documentation must a therapist prepare?*

- An individual report of the evaluation he or she conducted as a member of the IEP team.

- Relevant information and recommendations for a student's IEP as an IEP team member.

- A treatment plan for each child he or she serves.

- A supervision policy for OTAs and PTAs.

- In addition, an OT must document the child's status periodically and prepare a report after the child discontinues therapy.

As good practice, the therapist will write progress notes; document supervision of therapy assistants; keep records of treatment sessions; and keep records of phone contacts with parents, physicians, and other providers. The OT and PT contribute information on the amount of progress the student shows in meeting IEP goals. There is no requirement for each service provider on the IEP team to send a progress report to parents. When services are reimbursed by insurance, additional documentation is usually required.

2. *How long must therapists keep documentation?*
School districts may keep documentation classified as behavioral records no longer than one year after a pupil is no longer enrolled unless the pupil consents in writing to a longer period of record retention. The law does not specify how long a school should retain patient health care records. Districts may need documentation related to IEPs and Medicaid billing for up to five years. Local school board policy addresses records retention.

3. *How should a therapist write a treatment plan?*
In a treatment plan, the therapist typically describes the child's disability, medical diagnosis, contraindications to therapy, related IEP goal(s), therapy goals, and the equipment and personnel needed for interventions. Sample treatment plan formats are in Appendix B. Therapists may develop their own formats according to their plans to intervene. Therapists may change treatment plans as needed.

Other Practice Issues

1. *How is school-based occupational therapy and physical therapy different from clinical therapy?*
School-based therapy differs from clinical therapy in several aspects. Therapists provide service in school if a child requires it to benefit from special education. The emphasis in school therapy is to enable the child to participate in academic and non-academic activities within school environments. In a hospital or other medical facility, therapists typically provide interventions to remediate an acute or chronic medical problem or promote development. Clinical therapy also includes rehabilitation following a catastrophic illness or injury. Rehabilitation typically includes intensive services for several weeks or months to enable an individual to return to the community.

Therapists provide intervention in school only after an IEP team determines that a child has a disability and needs special education and occupational therapy or physical therapy. In a clinical model, therapists typically provide intervention that a physician requests.

2. *Can a therapist delegate procedures like brushing or range of motion to teachers or other school staff?*
   An OT may delegate occupational therapy to an OTA based upon the assistant's education, training, and experience. Wisconsin law does not allow anyone who is not an OT or an OTA to claim to render occupational therapy. (s. 448.03 (f)(g), Wis. Stats.)

   A PT may delegate a therapy procedure to a PTA based on the assistant's education, training, and experience. Wisconsin law requires that any physical therapy that someone other than the PT or PTA provides must be under the direct, on-premise supervision of the PT. (PT 5.02, Wis. Admin Code)

   OTs and PTs should not delegate direct therapy procedures that require the skills, knowledge, experience, training, and judgment of a therapist or assistant to teachers or other school staff. There are some school activities in which the roles and responsibilities of therapists and teachers coincide. For example, sitting in the classroom, writing, eating, and moving through the school are part of the child's school day. Both therapists and educators may have a role in helping the child increase his or her participation in these school activities. Therapists provide indirect service by collaborating with school staff to adapt materials, provide assistive technology, or integrate a skill learned during therapy into the classroom.

3. *Will Medicaid pay for occupational therapy and physical therapy that a school district provides as a related service on the child's IEP?*
   Yes, if the school meets the following requirements: the child must be eligible for Medicaid; the service must be medically necessary; the school or CESA must be a certified provider; the OT and PT must hold a DPI license and the parents must give written consent for the school to bill Medicaid. The Medicaid fiscal agent can provide schools with complete certification and billing information.

4. *Can therapists work with small groups of children?*
   Yes. Therapists provide service to small groups of children when that method of service delivery meets the unique needs of each child in the group. Small group intervention frequently occurs in early childhood classrooms. If the therapist plans to work with children in a small group, he or she should inform parents of the delivery method.

5. *Can a child receive direct physical therapy or occupational therapy under Section 504 without receiving special education?*
    Yes. A child can receive direct occupational therapy or physical therapy under Section 504 without receiving special education. Schools receive no state or federal reimbursement for services they provide under Section 504.

6. *If a child is enrolled in a private school, can he or she still receive occupational therapy or physical therapy as a related service?*
    A child who is enrolled in a private school by his or her parents may receive occupational therapy or physical therapy as a related service if these are services the child needs to benefit from special education, and if the school district agrees to provide these services to parentally placed private school students.

7. *May school OTs and school PTs provide services to children who do not have disabilities or have not been referred for a special education evaluation?*
    An OT or PT may provide services that are likely to improve occupational performance or functional movement for all students in a school. In educational terminology, this approach is called a universal intervention. It frequently takes the form of providing personnel development for teachers. If a school wants to provide targeted occupational therapy or physical therapy to children outside of the IEP team process, the school should consider

    *   licensure rules that require evaluation prior to providing service.

    *   licensure rules that require physician referral.

    *   parental informed consent.

    *   the possibility of an IDEA complaint.

    *   the provision of therapy to children without IEPs who need clinical services.

    *   limitations on the use of state and federal aid for occupational therapy and physical therapy that are not driven by IEPs.

Recruitment

1. *How can a school district obtain occupational therapy or physical therapy?*
    A district can obtain the services of an OT, a PT, an OTA, or a PTA by hiring the therapist or assistant on staff; contracting with a CESA or CCDEB; forming a 66:30 agreement with another agency to share therapy; or contracting with a hospital, clinic, private agency, individual therapist or individual assistant.

2. *What should a district do if it cannot find a therapist?*
    The district should try the following strategies.

    - Advertise the therapist position in the local newspapers and professional therapy journals and newsletters.

    - Post the position at colleges and universities that train therapists. Contact information for the training institutions are in Appendix A.

    - Seek a contract for a therapist through a CESA, 66:30 agreement, private agency, hospital, clinic, or public health agency.

    - Document all attempts to hire a therapist or contract for the service.

    - Notify the parents in writing about any interruption in therapy. Explain the steps being taken to hire or contract for the service.

    - Enlist the support of parents to notify the district of any therapist, agency, or hospital that may be able to provide the therapy.

    - If parents locate a therapist to serve their child, contact the therapist to arrange a contract between the therapist and the district, exploring whether the therapist has time to serve other students.

    - Arrange for transportation to and from therapy at a hospital or agency or offer to reimburse parents for transportation costs.

    - Provide therapy before or after school hours and on weekends at a hospital or agency.

    - Inform the parents periodically through letters, telephone calls, and group meetings about the good faith efforts of the district to obtain the therapist.

3. *What is a reasonable salary for therapists and assistant therapists?*
    Salaries for therapists vary throughout the state and depend on availability, experience, and labor agreements. Rates for contracted services are usually higher than staff salary rates. The teacher salary schedule may not offer competitive salaries for therapists. Districts may find that availability and competition with health care agencies governs salary ranges for therapists. A district can get information about local salaries by contacting other school districts, CESAs, hospitals and clinics in the region.

4. *How much supervisory time does the law require of a therapist if the district hires a full-time assistant?*
    The ratio of a therapist's FTE to an assistant's FTE is one to two. If the district hires a full-time assistant, the therapist must work at least .50 FTE. Under close supervision, the therapist must have daily, direct contact on the premises with the assistant. Under general supervision, the therapist must

have direct contact with the assistant at least once every 14 calendar days, providing on-site reevaluation of each child's therapy a minimum of one time per calendar month or every tenth day of therapy, whichever is sooner.

Licensing Issues

1. *Can a district hire a new graduate or someone who is waiting to take a professional board examination or waiting for the results of such an exam?*
   Yes, if that individual meets licensing requirements.

   - A graduate OT and OTA must have a temporary license from the Department of Regulation and Licensing (DRL) to practice. Practice during this period requires consultation with a licensed OT who shall at least once a month endorse the activities of the person holding the temporary license.

   - A graduate PT and PTA must have a temporary license from DRL to practice. Practice under a temporary license may not exceed 9 months. The PT must provide direct, immediate, and on-site supervision for the graduate PT or graduate PTA.

   - All therapy personnel must apply for a license from DPI, which will grant a one-year, provisional license until DRL issues a regular license.

2. *What if the OT, PT, OTA or PTA fails the licensure examination?*
   The individual cannot practice occupational therapy or physical therapy.

3. *What is an entry-level OT?*
   Entry-level refers to a person who has no demonstrated experience in a specific position, such as new graduate, a person new to the position, or a person in a new setting with no previous experience in the area of practice.

4. *Does DPI require specific continuing education for OT and PT license renewal?*
   No. PTs and PTAs must have current licenses from the DRL. Continuing education requirements for renewal of PT and PTA licenses are specified in Chapter PT 9, Wis. Admin Code. OTs and OTAs must have current licenses from DRL. Continuing education requirements for renewal of occupational therapy and OTA licenses under DRL are specified in Chapter OT 3, Wis. Admin Code.

Appendix A

Organizations

10

National Associations

American Occupational Therapy Association (AOTA)
(301) 652-AOTA (2682)
(301) 652-7711 (FAX)
(800) 377-8555 (TDD)
(800) SAY-AOTA (Member Line)
(301) 652-6611 (Voice Mail)
http://www.aota.org/

American Physical Therapy Association (APTA)
(703) 684-APTA (2782)
(703) 684-7343 (FAX)
(703) 683-6748 (TDD)
(800) 999-2782
http://www.apta.org/

The Association for Persons with Severe Handicaps (TASH)
(202) 540-9020
(202) 540-9019 (FAX)
http://www.healthfinder.gov/orgs/HR1486.htm

Council for Exceptional Children (CEC)
(888) 232-7733
(703) 264-9494 (FAX)
(866) 915-5000(TTY)
http://www.cec.sped.org//AM/Template.cfm?Section=Home

National Association of State Directors of Special Education
(703) 519-3800
(703) 519-3808 (FAX)
nasdse.org

National Board for Certification in Occupational Therapy (NBCOT)
(301) 990-7979
(301) 869-8492 (FAX)
http://www.nbcot.org/

National Dissemination Center for Children with Disabilities
NICHCY
(800) 695-0285 (V/TTY)
(202) 884-8200 (V/TTY)
(202)884-8441 (fax)
nichcy@aed.org
www.nichcy.org

RESNA: Rehabilitation Engineering and Assistive Technology Society of North America
(703) 524-6686
(703) 524-6630 (FAX)
http://resna.org/

ABLEDATA
(800) 227-0216.
http://www.abledata.com/

Disability.gov
Connecting the Disability Community to Information and Opportunities
https://www.disability.gov

State Organizations

Arc Wisconsin
(877) 272-8400
http://www.arc-wisconsin.org/

Autism Society of Wisconsin
(920) 558-4602
WI only: Toll-free 1-888-4-AUTISM (1-888-428-8476)
asw@asw4autism.org
http://www.asw4autism.org/

CHADD (Children with Attention Deficit Disorder)
http://www.chadd.org/

Family Assistance Center for Education, Training and Support
Wisconsin FACETS
(877) 374-4677 (Toll-free)
(414) 374-4655 (FAX)
(414) 374-4635 (TDD)
wifacets@wifacets.org
www.wifacets.org

Family Village
Clearinghouse of information for families of children with disabilities
Waisman Center
University of Wisconsin-Madison
http://www.familyvillage.wisc.edu/

Learning Disabilities Association of Wisconsin
ldainfo@LDAwisconsin.com
http://www.ldawisconsin.com/

Muscular Dystrophy Association (MDA)
http://www.mda.org/locate/

National Alliance on Mental Illness
NAMI Wisconsin Inc
(608)268-6000
(800)236-2988
www.namiwisconsin.org

United Cerebral Palsy of Southeastern Wis. Inc.
(414) 329-4500
(414) 329-4511 (TTY)
(414) 329-4510 (FAX)
Toll Free: 888-482-7739
info@ucpsew.org
http://www.ucpsew.org/

Wisconsin Occupational Therapy Association (WOTA)
(608) 287-1606
(800) 728-1992 (members only)
(608) 287-1608 (FAX)
wota@execpc.com
www.wota.net

Wisconsin Physical Therapy Association (WPTA)
(608) 221-9191
Consumer Hotline Toll Free: (866) FOR-MYPT (367-6978)
(608) 221-9697 (FAX)
wpta@wpta.org
http://www.wpta.org/

Federal Agencies

Department of Education
Office of Civil Rights (OCR)
U.S. Department of Education
Hotline: 1-800-421-3481
http://www2.ed.gov/about/offices/list/ocr/index.html

Office of Civil Rights, Chicago Office (Region V)
U. S. Department of Education
(312) 730-1560
(312) 730-1576 (FAX)
(312) 730-1609 (TDD)
OCR.Chicago@ed.gov

Office of Special Education Programs (OSEP)
U.S. Department of Education
(800) 872-5327
(800) 437-0833 (TTY)
http://www2.ed.gov/about/offices/list/osers/osep/index.html

Office of Special Education and Rehabilitative Services (OSERS)
U.S. Department of Education
(800) 872-5327
(800) 437-0833 (TTY)
http://www2.ed.gov/about/offices/list/osers/index.html

U.S. Government Printing Office
DC metro area   (202) 512-1800
toll free   (866) 512-1800
fax   (202) 512-.2104
gpo@custhelp.com
http://www.gpo.gov/

State Agencies

State of Wisconsin Home Page
Includes Wisconsin state agencies
http://www.state.wi.us/state/index.html

Department of Administration
Document Sales & Distribution
Phone Orders: (608) 266-3358, (800) 362-7253, or (608) 264-9419
(608) 261-8150 (FAX)
docsales@doa.state.wi.us
State of Wisconsin Document Sales Catalog
http://www.doa.state.wi.us/docview.asp?docid=6590&locid=2

Department of Children and Families (DCF)
(608) 267-3905
(608) 266-6836 (FAX)
dcfweb@wisconsin.gov
http://dcf.wi.gov/default.htm

Department of Commerce
(608) 266-1018
http://www.commerce.state.wi.us/

Department of Health Services (DHS)
(608) 266-1865
http://dhs.wisconsin.gov/

DHS Telephone Hotlines
http://dhs.wisconsin.gov/data/hotline.asp

Bureau of Health Care Financing (Medical Assistance)
(608) 266-2522
(800) 362-3002
(608) 266-4279 (TDD)
dhswebmaildhcf@wisconsin.govhttp://dhs.wisconsin.gov/medicaid/index.htm

School-Based Services (SBS)
SBS/MAC Policy (608) 266-9815, Gregory.Dimiceli@wi.gov
SBS/MAC Fiscal (608) 266-3802, Steve.Milioto@wi.gov

Division of Health Care Access and Accountability
EDI Department
(608) 221-9036
wiedi@dhfs.state.wi.us

Long Term Care and Support Services
http://dhs.wisconsin.gov/programs/ltc.htm
Autism Services: http://dhs.wisconsin.gov/bdds/clts/autism/
Birth to 3 Program: http://dhs.wisconsin.gov/bdds/birthto3/index.htm
Center for People with Intellectual Disabilities: http://dhs.wisconsin.gov/Disabilities/dd_ctrs/index.htm
Children's Long Term Support Waivers: http://dhs.wisconsin.gov/bdds/clts/index.htm
Children with Special Health Care Needs: http://dhs.wisconsin.gov/health/children/
Family Support : http://dhs.wisconsin.gov/bdds/fsp/
Katie Beckett: http://dhs.wisconsin.gov/bdds/kbp/

First Step (Birth to Six Information and Referral)
(800) 642-STEP (7837)

WisTech
Assistive Technology Information Network
Office of Independence and Employment
(608) 267-9091
(608) 267-9880 (TTY)
(608) 266-3386 (FAX)
ralph.pelkey@dhs.wisconsin.gov
sarah.lincoln@dhs.wisconsin.gov
http://dhs.wisconsin.gov/disabilities/wistech/whatiswistech.htm

Department of Public Instruction (DPI)
(608) 266-3390
(800) 441-4563
(608) 267-2427 (TDD)
(608) 267-3746 (FAX Special Education)
http://dpi.wi.gov/
(608) 266-1027 Licenses
http://dpi.wi.gov/sped/tm-specedtopics.html (Special Education Index)

Department of Regulation and Licensing (DRL)
(608) 266-2811
(877) 617-1565
http://drl.wi.gov/

Occupational Therapists Affiliated Credentialing Board (OTACB)
http://drl.wi.gov/board_detail.asp?boardid=44&locid=0

Physical Therapy Examining Board (PTEB)
http://drl.wi.gov/board_detail.asp?boardid=47&locid=0

Department of Transportation (DOT)
Transportation Safety
(608) 266-0402
http://www.dot.wisconsin.gov/about/
Phone Guide: http://www.dot.wisconsin.gov/about/contacts/phoneguide.htm#S
School buses   (608) 267-3154
Seat belts/car seats   (608) 267-7520
Safety schools   (608) 266-2237
Driver license information   (608) 266-2353
Equipment   (608) 266-0094

Department of Workforce Development (DWD)
Civil Rights Bureau
Equal Rights Division
http://dwd.wisconsin.gov/

Madison Office
(608) 266-6860
(608) 267-4592 (FAX)
(608) 264-8752 (TTY)

Milwaukee Office
(414) 227-4384
(414) 227-4084 (FAX)
(414) 227-4081 (TTY)

Division of Vocational Rehabilitation (Transition)
(800) 442-3477 (Toll Free)
(608) 266-1133 (FAX)
(888) 877-5939 (TTY)
dvr@dwd.wisconsin.gov
http://dwd.wisconsin.gov/dvr/

University and Technical College Programs

Accredited Occupational Therapy Programs
http://www.aota.org/Students/Schools/EntryLevelOT/38119.aspx#wi

Accredited Occupational Therapy Assistant Programs
http://www.aota.org/Students/Schools/EntryLevelOT/38117.aspx

Accredited Occupational Therapy Doctoral Level Programs
http://www.aota.org/Students/Schools/EntryLevelOT/Doctoral.aspx

Accredited Physical Therapist Education Programs
http://apps.apta.org/Custom/wstemplate.cfm?cfml=accreditedschools/Index.cfm&cfmltitle=Accredited%20PT%20and%20PTA%20Programs&process=1&state=WI&type=PT&&fromStudentMap=1

Accredited Physical Therapist Assistant Education Programs
http://apps.apta.org/Custom/wstemplate.cfm?cfml=accreditedschools/Index.cfm&cfmltitle=Accredited%20PT%20and%20PTA%20Programs&process=1&state=WI&type=PTA&&fromStudentMap=1

Post Professional Physical Therapist Programs
http://www.apta.org/PostprofessionalDegree/GraduatePrograms/

Carroll University
Physical Therapy Program
(262) 650-4915
www.carrollu.edu

Concordia University
Occupational Therapy Program
(262) 243-4429
www.cuw.edu

Department of Physical Therapy
(262) 243-4433
www.cuw.edu

Marquette University
Department of Physical Therapy
(414) 288-7194
www.marquette.edu/chs/pt

Mount Mary College
Occupational Therapy Program
(414)-256-1246
www.mtmary.edu/ot.htm

University of Wisconsin-La Crosse
Occupational Therapy Program
(608) 785-6620
www.uwlax.edu/ot/

Physical Therapy Program
(608) 785-8470
http://www.uwlax.edu/pt/

University of Wisconsin-Madison
Occupational Therapy Program
(608) 262-2936
www.education.wisc.edu/kinesiology/ot/
welcome/default.aspx

Physical Therapy Program
(608) 263-7131
http://www.orthorehab.wisc.edu/pt

University of Wisconsin-Milwaukee
Occupational Therapy Program
(414) 229-4713
www.uwm.edu/chs/academics/occupational_
therapy/

Physical Therapy Program
(414) 229-3265
www.uwm.edu

Blackhawk Technical College
Physical Therapist Assistant Program
(608) 757-7698
www.blackhawk.edu

Chippewa Valley Technical College
Physical Therapist Assistant Program
(715) 833-6417
www.cvtc.edu

Fox Valley Technical College
Occupational Therapy Assistant Program
(920) 735-5645 or (920) 831-4333
www.fvtc.edu/public/

Gateway Technical College
Physical Therapist Assistant Program
(262) 564-2482
www.gtc.edu

Madison Area Technical College
Occupational Therapy Assistant Program
(608) 246-6065
www.matcmadison.edu

Milwaukee Area Technical College
Occupational Therapy Assistant Program
(414) 297-6882
http://matc.edu/student/offerings/otasst.html

Physical Therapist Assistant Program
(414) 297-8078
http://matc.edu/student/offerings/phyasst.html

Northeast Wisconsin Technical College
Occupational Therapy Assistant Program
(920) 498-5543
www.nwtc.edu

Western Wisconsin Technical College
Occupational Therapy Assistant Program
(608) 785-9585
www.westerntc.edu

Physical Therapist Assistant Program
(608) 785-9598
www.westerntc.edu

Wisconsin Indianhead Technical College-Ashland Campus
Occupational Therapy Assistant Program
(715) 682-4591
www.witc.edu

Appendix B

Sample Occupational Therapy or Physical Therapy Treatment Plans

Child's Name		Date of Birth	
Physician		Medical Information	
Last Evaluation	Disability	Annual IEP date	Amount and Frequency
Target IEP Goals			
Therapy objectives	Objective 1	Objective 2	Objective 3
Level of function			
Contraindications to therapy or other participation			
Planned interventions			
Indirect services plan			
Coordination with community therapist or other programs			
Delegation to assistant			
Progress / /			
Progress / /			
Progress / /			

Sample Occupational Therapy Treatment Plan

Child's name: Date of Birth: Age:

Physician: Disability:

Contraindications:

Date of plan:

Target goal and objectives

Identify annual goals from IEP that occupational therapy supports.

Identify specific treatment goals in occupational therapy and baseline measurements.

     Performance area: (ADL, work or productive activities, or play/leisure)

     Performance components: (Sensorimotor, cognitive, or psychosocial)

     Performance contexts: (Temporal, environment)

Intervention

Identify approaches, procedures and activities, and location of services.

Indirect services

Identify implementer, collaboration strategies, and proposed meeting schedule.

Delegation to OTA

Identify portion of treatment plan, level and frequency of supervision.

Coordination with therapist outside school setting

Identify plan to share treatment plan and progress notes. Attach copy of parental consent for release of information. Document communication.

Progress

Identify method and content of progress monitoring

Sample progress chart

Expected Outcome	Initial status	Date/ Status	Date/ Status	Date/ Status	Date/ Status	Date/ Status

Sample Physical Therapy Treatment Plan

Child's name: Date of Birth: Age:

Physician: Disability:

Contraindications:

Date of plan:

Present level of motoric/functional performance

Target goal and objectives

Identify annual goals from IEP that physical therapy supports.

Identify specific treatment goals in physical therapy and baseline measurements.

Intervention

Identify strategies, procedures and activities, and location of services.

Indirect services

Identify implementer, collaboration strategies, and proposed meeting schedule.

Delegation to PTA

Identify portion of treatment plan, level and frequency of supervision.

Coordination with therapist outside school setting

Identify plan to share treatment plan and progress notes. Attach copy of parental consent for release of information. Document communication.

Progress

Identify method and content of progress monitoring

Sample progress chart

Expected Outcome	Initial status	Date/ Status	Date/ Status	Date/ Status	Date/ Status	Date/ Status

Sample Occupational Therapy Treatment Plan

Child's name: _____ Date: _____

Teacher: _____ Birth date:

_____

LEA name: _____Chron. age: _____ yrs._____mo.

IEP goal:_____

_____

_____

Target occupational performance:_____

_____

_____

Context:_____

_____

Outcome category: _____ Academic learning _____ Play/leisure _____ Employment

_____ Social participation _____ ADL/Community skills

Intervention approach: ___ create/promote ___ establish/restore ___maintain

___modify/compensate ___ prevent

Intervention will address ____client factors ___activity demands ___context and environments

_____ performance skills ___ performance patterns

Performance factors:

Enabling factors: _____ Concerns:_____

_____ _____

_____ _____

_____ _____

_____ _____

Intervention implementation:

Collaborative consultation: amount/frequency_____location_____duration_____

Implementer: ___ teacher ___aide ___ family ___other_____

Specific interventions: _____

_____

Training and Verification Strategies:_____

Proposed Meeting Schedule: ___ weekly ___ bimonthly ____monthly ____other_____

Location of Meeting:_____

Individual direct service: amount/frequency_____location_____duration_____

Implementer: ___ OT ___OTA

Specific interventions: _____

_____

_____

Method for Documentation of Performance:

Behavior to be observed: _____

Natural environment for observation: _____

Measurement/data to be collected: _____

By whom: _____ Frequency: _____

Criterion for successful performance:_____

_____

Sample Physical Therapy Treatment Plan

DeForest School District, reprinted with permission.

Student: DOB/Age: Therapist(s):
Parent(s):   Phone: Physician:
School: Grade: Teacher:
Frequency: IEP due: Date of 3-year re-evaluation:
Date of plan:

IEP Objectives:

Current status of objectives/function:

Medical Information:

Precautions:

Recommendations from IEP Team
- ❑ Ambulation/gait training
- ❑ Wheelchair mobility
- ❑ Transfer training
- ❑ Gross motor skills
- ❑ Positioning

- ❑ Posture
- ❑ Sensory motor skills
- ❑ Eye-hand coordination
- ❑ Balance
- ❑ Strength/stability

- ❑ Motor planning skills
- ❑ Ball skills
- ❑ Equipment

Treatment Strategies

Intervention
- ❑ Individual
- ❑ Small group
- ❑ PE class
- ❑ Therapy room
- ❑ Classroom

Ambulation
- ❑ Even surfaces
- ❑ Uneven surfaces
- ❑ Steps
- ❑ Distance/speed
- ❑ Independently
- ❑ Assistive devices

Balance
- ❑ Balance beam
- ❑ Single limb stance
- ❑ Therapy balls
- ❑ Changing directions
- ❑ Obstacle course

Mat skills
- ❑ Roll
- ❑ All 4's
- ❑ Stand to sit
- ❑ Sit to stand
- ❑ Tall kneel

Strengthening
- ❑ Overall
- ❑ Lower extremities
- ❑ Trunk

Wheelchair mobility
- ❑ Independent propulsion
- ❑ Hallways
- ❑ Doorways
- ❑ In crowds
- ❑ Ramps

High level locomotor skills
- ❑ Skipping
- ❑ Running
- ❑ Galloping
- ❑ Hopping

Jumping skills
- ❑ Jump rope
- ❑ Jump high and long
- ❑ Jump down
- ❑ Consecutive

Climbing
- ❑ Playground equip
- ❑ Stairs
- ❑ Over obstacles

Ball skills
- ❑ Kicking
- ❑ Throwing
- ❑ Catching
- ❑ Dribbling

Posture/positioning
- ❑ Classroom equipment
- ❑ Sitting posture
- ❑ Standing activities
- ❑ Assistive devices

Eye-hand coordination
- ❑ Batting
- ❑ Racket activities

Sensory motor
- ❑ Swing
- ❑ Scooter board
- ❑ Therapy balls
- ❑ Proprioceptive input
- ❑ Vestibular input
- ❑ Tactile input

Classroom Recommendations:
- ❑ Modified seating
- ❑ Sensory inputs
- ❑ Strengthening activities
- ❑ Other

Appendix C

Pediatric Physical Therapy Assessment Tools

Body Structure and Function

Assessment	Description	Resource
30-Second Walk Test	Describes the distance students without disabilities ages 6-13 years walk in 30 seconds.	Knutson, L., P. Schimmel, and A. Ruff. 1999. "Standard Task Measurement for Mobility: Thirty-Second Walk Test." *Pediatric Physical Therapy* 11(4):183–90.
30-Second Walk Test – Age Expansion	Expands by age the 30-second walk test norms for children ages 5-17 years.	Knutson, L., B. Bushman, J. C. Young, and G. Ward. 2009. "Age Expansion of the Thirty Second Walk Test Norms for Children." *Pediatric Physical Therapy* 21(3):235–43.
6-Minute Walk Test (6MWT)	Measures exercise capacity in children ages 4-11 years who have chronic cardiac or respiratory disease.	Lammers, A. E., A. A. Hislop, Y. Flynn, S. G. Haworth. 2007. "The 6-minute walk test: normal values for children of 4-11 years of age." Department of Paediatric Cardiology, Great Ormond Street Hospital for Children, Great Ormond Street, London WC1N 3JH, UK) http://adc.bmj.com/cgi/content/abstract/93/6/464
Energy Expenditure Index	Quantifies and compares walking energy expenditure for children and adolescents.	Rose, J., J G. Gamble, J. Lee, R. Lee, and W. L. Haskell. 1991. "The energy expenditure index: a method to quantitate and compare walking energy expenditure for children and adolescents." *Journal of Pediatric Orthopedics* 11:571–77.
Faces Pain Scale-Revised	Self-assesses pain severity for children ages 4-16 years.	Hicks CL, CL.von Baeyer, P. Spafford, I. van Korlaar and B. Goodenough. 2001. "The Faces Pain Scale - Revised: Toward a common metric in pediatric pain measurement." *Pain* 93:173–83. http://painsourcebook.ca/docs/pps92.html
Functional Reach Test	Examines dynamic balance in children ages 3-5 years.	Norris, R.A., E. Wilder, and J. Norton. 2008. "The Functional Reach Test in 3- to5- Year-Old Children Without Disabilities." *Pediatric Physical Therapy* 20(1):47–52.
Modified Time Up and Go (Modified TUG)	Measures anticipatory standing balance and walking.	Williams, E. N. et al. 2005. *Developmental Medicine and Child Neurology* 47:518–24.
Motor Function Measure Scale for	Measures motor function for individuals with neuromuscular	Berard, C., C. Payan, I. Hodgkinson, J. Fermanian. 2005. "A motor function

Assessment	Description	Resource
Neuromuscular Diseases (MFM)	diseases ages 6-62 years.	measure scale for neuromuscular diseases." The MFM Collaborative Study Group. *Neuromuscular Disorders* 15:463–70. http://www.mfm-nmd.org/upload/File/MFM%20article%20Neuro%20muscular%20disorders%202005.pdf
Pediatric Balance Scale	Measures the performance of children developing typically.	Franjoine, M.R.,N. Darr, S. Held, K. Kott, and B. Young. 2010. "The Performance of Children Developing Typically on the Pediatric Balance Scale." *Pediatric Physical Therapy* 22(4): 350-359.
Pediatric Berg Balance Scale	Measures functional balance for school-age children with mild to moderate motor impairments.	Franjoine, M.R., J. Gurther, and M. J. Taylor. 2003. "Pediatric Balance Scale: A Modified Version of the Berg Balance Scale for the School-Age Child with Mild to Moderate Motor Impairment." *Pediatric Physical Therapy* 15(2):114–20.
Pediatric Clinical Test of Sensory Integration and Balance (P-CTSIB or Foam and Dome)	Provides information about the ability to stand upright under several sensory conditions.	Crowe, T. K., J. C. Dietz, P. K. Richardson, and S. L. Westcott. 1994. "Test-Retest Reliability of the Pediatric Clinical Test of Sensory Interaction for Balance." *Physical and Occupational Therapy in Pediatrics* 14:1.
Standardized Walking Obstacle Course (SWOC)	Measures functional ambulation for children with and without disabilities who walk without an assistive device.	Held, S., K. M. Kott, and B.L. Young. 2006. "Standardized Walking Obstacle Course (SWOC): Reliability and Validity of a New Functional Measurement Tool for Children." *Pediatric Physical Therapy* 18(1):23–30.
Test of Gross Motor Development-2 (TGMD-2)	Measures twelve gross motor skills ages 3 -10 years to identify children who are significantly behind their peers in gross motor development.	Ulrich, D.A. 2000. "The Test of Gross Motor Development" 2nd ed. *PRO-ED, Inc.* 8700 Shoal Creek Boulevard Austin, Texas 78757-6897 http://www.pef.uni-lj.si/srp_gradiva/tgm.pdf
Timed Up and Down Stairs (TUDS)	Measures functional mobility for children with and without cerebral palsy ages 8-14 years.	Zaino, C., V.G Marchese, and S. L. Westcott. 2004. "Timed Up and Down Stairs Test: Preliminary Reliability and Validity of a New Measure of Functional Mobility." *Pediatric Physical Therapy* 16(2):90–8.
Timed Up and Go (TUG)	Measures mobility in individuals who are able to walk on their own.	*Developmental Medicine and Child Neurology.* 2005. 47:518–24. http://www.fallprevention.ri.gov/Module3/sld007.htm
Walking Speeds Standards	Provides walking speeds standards for students in	David, K., and M. Sullivan. 2005. "Expectations for Walking Speeds:

Assessment	Description	Resource
	elementary school along hallways/50 ft. paths.	Standards for Students in Elementary Schools." *Pediatric Physical Therapy* 17(2): 120–27.

Activity

Assessment	Description	Resource
Bruininks-Osteretsky Test of Motor Proficiency, Second Edition (BOT-2)	Assesses motor functioning of children ages 4-21 years in areas of fine motor control, manual coordination, body coordination, strength and agility.	Pearson, Attn: Customer Service, 19500 Bulverde Road, San Antonio, TX 78259-3701; Phone: 800.627.7271; Fax: 800.232.1223. ClinicalCustomerSupport@Pearson.com
Functional Independence Measure (WEE FIM II)	Measures the need for assistance and the severity of disability in children ages 6 months - 7 years. Eighteen items measure functional performance in three domains.	Uniform Data System for Medical Rehabilitation, 270 Northpointe Parkway, Suite 300, Amherst, NY 14228; phone: 716-817-7800 (Mon-Fri, 8:30 a.m.-5:30 p.m. EST); fax: 716-568-0037. info@udsmr.org
Gross Motor Function Measure (GMFM)	Evaluates change in gross motor function in children with cerebral palsy and describes current level of motor function.	Bjornson, K. F, C. S. Graubert, V. L Buford, et al. 1998. "Validity of the Gross Motor Function Measure." *Pediatric Physical Therapy* 10(2):43–47.
Gross Motor Function Measure (GMFM) for Children with Down Syndrome	Determines validity of the GMFM for evaluating motor function in children with Down Syndrome.	Russell, D., R. Palisano, S. Walter, et al. 1998. *Developmental Medicine and Child Neurology* 40:693–701.
Gross Motor Function Measure (GMFM) for Children with OI	Determines reliability of the GMFM for children with Osteogenesis Imperfecta.	Ruck-Gibis, J., H. Plotkin, J. Hanley, and S. Wood-Dauphinee, 2001. "Reliability of the Gross Motor Function Measure for Children with Osteogenesis Imperfecta." *Pediatric Physical Therapy* 13(1):10–17.
Gross Motor Function Measure (GMFM-88 and GMFM-66)	Measures change in gross motor function in children with cerebral palsy ages 5 months - 16 years. Also valid for assessment of children with Down Syndrome and children recovering from TBI.	Russell, D., P. L. Rosenbaum, L. M. Avery, and M. Lane. 2002. Wiley, Customer Care Center - Consumer Accounts, 10475 Crosspoint Blvd., Indianapolis, IN 46256; Phone: 877-762-2974; Fax: 800-597-3299; http://www.wiley.com/WileyCDA/WileyTitle/productCd-1898683301.html
Movement Assessment Battery for Children, Second Edition (MABC-2)	Screens/identifies motor competence for children in three age ranges: 3-6; 7-10; and 11-16 years. Eight items tested for each age group in three areas: manual dexterity, ball skills, and static and dynamic	Pearson, Attn: Customer Service, 19500 Bulverde Road, San Antonio, TX 78259-3701; Phone: 800.627.7271; Fax: 800.232.1223. ClinicalCustomerSupport@Pearson.com http://www.psychcorp.co.uk/index.aspx

Assessment	Description	Resource
	balance.	
Peabody Developmental Motor Scales (PDMS-2), Second Edition	Measures gross and fine motor skills from birth-6 years.	Pearson, Attn: Customer Service, 19500 Bulverde Road, San Antonio, TX 78259-3701; Phone: 800.627.7271; Fax: 800.232.1223. ClinicalCustomerSupport@Pearson.com

Activity and Participation Tests

Assessment	Description	Resource
Pediatric Evaluation of Disability Inventory (PEDI)	Measures capability and performance of functional activities in self care, mobility, and social function in children from 6 months - 7.5 years.	Pearson, Attn: Customer Service, 19500 Bulverde Road, San Antonio, TX 78259-3701; Phone: 800.627.7271; Fax: 800.232.1223. ClinicalCustomerSupport@Pearson.com
School Function Assessment (SFA)	Measures participation in school-related activities, activity performance, and the need for assistance or accommodations for students grades K-6.	Pearson, Attn: Customer Service, 19500 Bulverde Road, San Antonio, TX 78259-3701; Phone: 800.627.7271; Fax: 800.232.1223. ClinicalCustomerSupport@Pearson.com

Activity and Participation Tests—Transition

Assessment	Description	Resource
Canadian Occupational Performance Measure (COPM)	Measures change in parents or student's self-perception of functional performance over time.	Contact Mary Law at lawm@mcmaster.ca 4th ed. May 2005.
Enderle-Severson Transition Rating Scale	Measures the needs, preferences, and interests of students with disabilities for transition post high school; for students with mild disabilities and for moderate to severe disabilities; and a form for parents.	ESTR Publications 1907 18th St. S, Moorhead MN 56560; 218-287-8477; Fax (218) 236-5199. www.estr.net

Participation Tests

Assessment	Description	Resource
Assessment of Life Habits (LIFE–H)	Measures social participation in eleven life habit categories.	Noreau, L., P. Fougeyrollas, and C. Vincent. 2002. "The LIFE-H: Assessment of the quality of social participation." *Technology and Disability* 14:113–18.
Children's Assessment of Participation and Enjoyment (CAPE) and Preference for Activity of Children (PAC)	Measures participation in leisure activities for ages 6-21 years.	Pearson, Attn: Customer Service 19500 Bulverde Road, San Antonio, TX 78259-3701; Phone: 800.627.7271; Fax: 800.232.1223. ClinicalCustomerSupport@Pearson.com
Pediatric Quality of Life Inventory (PedsQLTM)	Measures physical, emotional, social, and school function for four age band groups, ages 2-18 years.	J. W. Varni. Child Self Report at http://www.pedsql.org/pedsql13.html

Classification Systems

Assessment	Description	Resource
Gross Motor Function Classification System Expanded and Revised (GMFCS-E & R)	Classifies on five levels motor function for children with cerebral palsy. http://canchild-mgm.icreate3.esolutionsgroup.ca/en/GMFCS/resources/GMFCSER6-12.pdf	Palisano, R., P. Rosenbaum, D. Bartlett, and M. Livingston. 2007. CanChild Centre for Childhood Disability Research, McMaster University. Free to the public through the CanChild website: www.canchild.ca/en/
Manual Ability Classification System (MACS)	Classifies on five levels functional hand use for children with cerebral palsy.	Eliasson, A. C., L. Krumlinde Sundholm, B. Rösblad, E. Beckung, M. Arner, A. M. Öhrvall, and P. Rjosenbaum. 2006. *Developmental Medicine and Child Neurology* 48:549–54.

Program Evaluation

Assessment	Description	Resource
School Outcomes Measure (SOM)	Collects outcomes of children who receive school -based physical therapy and occupational therapy.	Arnold S.H. and I. R. McEwen. 2008. "Item Test Reliability and Responsiveness of the School Outcomes Measure (SOM)." *Physical and Occupational Therapy in Pediatrics* 28:59–77. SomResearch@ouhsc.edu http://www.ah.ouhsc.edu/somresearch/index.asp http://www.ah.ouhsc.edu/somresearch/adminGuide.pdf

Appendix D

Codes of Ethics

AOTA Occupational Therapy Code of Ethics and Ethics Standards

The *Occupational Therapy Code of Ethics and Ethics Standards* (2010) from the American Occupational Therapy Association defines the set of principles that apply to occupational therapy personnel at all levels. Because of the length of the document, it is not reprinted here but is available in the *American Journal of Occupational Therapy*, 64:6 and online at http://www.aota.org/Practitioners/Ethics/Docs.aspx.

APTA Code of Ethics for the Physical Therapist

American Physical Therapy Association. APTA HOD S06-09-07-12 [Amended HOD S06-00-12-23; HOD 06-91-05-05;HOD 06-87-11-17; American Physical Therapy Association w HOD 06-81-06-18; HOD 06-78-06-08; HOD 06-78-06-07; HOD 06-77-18-30; HOD 06-77-17-27; Initial HOD 06-73-13-24] [Standard]. Reprinted with permission.

Preamble

The Code of Ethics for the Physical Therapist (Code of Ethics) delineates the ethical obligations of all physical therapists as determined by the House of Delegates of the American Physical Therapy Association (APTA). The purposes of this Code of Ethics are to:

1. Define the ethical principles that form the foundation of physical therapist practice in patient/client management, consultation, education, research, and administration.
2. Provide standards of behavior and performance that form the basis of professional accountability to the public.
3. Provide guidance for physical therapists facing ethical challenges, regardless of their professional roles and responsibilities.
4. Educate physical therapists, students, other health care professionals, regulators, and the public regarding the core values, ethical principles, and standards that guide the professional conduct of the physical therapist.
5. Establish the standards by which the American Physical Therapy Association can determine if a physical therapist has engaged in unethical conduct.

No code of ethics is exhaustive nor can it address every situation. Physical therapists are encouraged to seek additional advice or consultation in install.ces where the guidance of the Code of Ethics may not be definitive.

This Code of Ethics is built upon the five roles of the physical therapist (management of patients/clients, consultation, education, research, and administration), the core values of the profession, and the multiple realms of ethical action (individual, organizational, and societal). Physical therapist practice is guided by a set of seven core values: accountability, altruism, compassion/caring, excellence, integrity, professional duty, and social responsibility. Throughout the document the primary core values that support specific principles are indicated in parentheses. Unless a specific role is indicated in the principle, the duties and obligations being delineated pertain to the five roles of the physical therapist. Fundamental to the Code of Ethics is the special obligation of physical therapists to empower, educate, and enable those with impairments, activity limitations, participation restrictions, and disabilities to facilitate greater independence, health, wellness, and enhanced quality of life.

Principles

Principle #1: Physical therapists shall respect the inherent dignity rights of all individuals. (Core Values: Compassion, Integrity)

1A. Physical therapists shall act in a respectful manner toward each person regardless of age, gender, race, nationality, religion, ethnicity, social or economic status, sexual orientation, health condition, or disability.

1B. Physical therapists shall recognize their personal biases and shall not discriminate against others in physical therapist practice, consultation, education, research, and administration.

Principle #2: Physical therapists shall be trustworthy and compassionate in addressing the rights and needs of patients/clients. Core Values: Altruism, Compassion, Professional Duty

2A. Physical therapists shall adhere to the core values of the profession and shall act in the best interests of patients/clients over the interests of the physical therapist.

2B. Physical therapists shall provide physical therapy services with compassionate and caring behaviors that incorporate the individual and cultural differences of patients/clients.

2C. Physical therapists shall provide the information necessary to allow patients or their surrogates to make informed decisions about physical therapy care or participation in clinical research.

2D. Physical therapists shall collaborate with patients/clients to empower them in decisions about their health care.

2E. Physical therapists shall protect confidential patient/client information and may disclose confidential information to appropriate authorities only when allowed or as required by law.

Principle #3: Physical therapists shall be accountable for making sound professional judgments. (Core Values: Excellence, Integrity)

3A. Physical therapists shall demonstrate independent and objective professional judgment in the patient's/client's best interest in all practice settings.

3B. Physical therapists shall demonstrate professional judgment informed by professional standards, evidence (including current literature and established best practice), practitioner experience, and patient/client values.

3C. Physical therapists shall make judgments within their scope of practice and level of expertise and shall communicate with, collaborate with, or refer to peers or other health care professionals when necessary.

3D. Physical therapists shall not engage in conflicts of interest that interfere with professional judgment.

3E. Physical therapists shall provide appropriate direction of and communication with physical therapist assistants and support personnel.

Principle #4: Physical therapists shall demonstrate integrity in their relationships with patients/clients, families, colleagues, students, research participants, other health care providers, employers, payers and the public. (Core Value: Integrity)

4A. Physical therapists shall provide truthful, accurate and relevant information and shall not make misleading representations.

4B. Physical therapists shall not exploit persons over whom they have supervisory, evaluative or other authority (e.g., patients/clients, students, supervisees, research participants, or employees).

4C. Physical therapists shall discourage misconduct by health care professionals and report illegal or unethical acts to the relevant authority, when appropriate.

4D. Physical therapists shall report suspected cases of abuse involving children or vulnerable adults to the appropriate authority, subject to law.

4E. Physical therapists shall not engage in any sexual relationship with any of their patients/clients, supervisees, or students.

4F. Physical therapists shall not harass anyone verbally, physically, emotionally, or sexually.

Principle #5: Physical therapists shall fulfill their legal and professional obligations. (Core Values: Professional Duty, Accountability)

5A. Physical therapists shall comply with applicable local, state, and federal laws and regulations.

5B. Physical therapists shall have primary responsibility for supervision of physical therapist assistants and support personnel.

5C. Physical therapists involved in research shall abide by accepted standards governing protection of research participants.

5D. Physical therapists shall encourage colleagues with physical, psychological, or substance-related impairments that may adversely impact their professional responsibilities to seek assistance or counsel.

5E. Physical therapists who have knowledge that a colleague is unable to perform their professional responsibilities with reasonable skill and safety shall report this information to the appropriate authority.

5F. Physical therapists shall provide notice and information about alternatives for obtaining care in the event the physical therapist terminates the provider relationship while the patient/client continues to need physical therapy services.

Principle #6: Physical therapists shall enhance their expertise through the lifelong acquisition and refinement of knowledge, skills, abilities, and professional behaviors. (Core Value: Excellence)

6A. Physical therapists shall achieve and maintain professional competence.

6B. Physical therapists shall take responsibility for their professional development based on critical self-assessment and reflection on changes in physical therapist practice, education, health care delivery, and technology.

6C. Physical therapists shall evaluate the strength of evidence and applicability of content presented during professional development activities before integrating the content or techniques into practice.

6D. Physical therapists shall cultivate practice environments that support professional development, lifelong learning, and excellence.

Principle #7: Physical therapists shall promote organizational behaviors and business practices that benefit patients/clients and society. (Core Values: Integrity, Accountability)

7A. Physical therapists shall promote practice environments that support autonomous and accountable professional judgments.

7B. Physical therapists shall seek remuneration as is deserved and reasonable for physical therapist services.

7C. Physical therapists shall not accept gifts or other considerations that influence or give an appearance of influencing their professional judgment.

7D. Physical therapists shall fully disclose any financial interest they have in products or services that they recommend to patients/clients.

7E. Physical therapists shall be aware of charges and shall ensure that documentation and coding for physical therapy services accurately reflect the nature and extent of the services provided.

7F. Physical therapists shall refrain from employment arrangements, or other arrangements, that prevent physical therapists from fulfilling professional obligations to patients/clients.

Principle #8: Physical therapists shall participate in efforts to meet the health needs of people locally, nationally, or globally. (Core Value: Social Responsibility)

8A. Physical therapists shall provide pro bono physical therapy services or support organizations that meet the health needs of people who are economically disadvantaged, uninsured, and underinsured.

8B. Physical therapists shall advocate to reduce health disparities and health care inequities, improve access to health care services, and address the health, wellness, and preventive health care needs of people.

8C. Physical therapists shall be responsible stewards of health care resources and shall avoid overutilization or underutilization of physical therapy services.

8D. Physical therapists shall educate members of the public about the benefits of physical therapy and the unique role of the physical therapist.

APTA Standards of Ethical Conduct for the Physical Therapist Assistant

American Physical Therapy Association. APTA HOD S06-09-20-18 [Amended HOD S06-00-13-24; HOD 06-91-06-07; Initial HOD 06-82-04-08] [Standard]

Preamble

The Standards of Ethical Conduct for the Physical Therapist Assistant (Standards of Ethical Conduct) delineate the ethical obligations of all physical therapist assistants as determined by the House of Delegates of the American Physical Therapy Association (APTA). The Standards of Ethical Conduct provide a foundation for conduct to which all physical therapist assistants shall adhere. Fundamental to the Standards of Ethical Conduct is the special obligation of physical therapist assistants to enable patients/clients to achieve greater independence, health and wellness, and enhanced quality of life.

No document that delineates ethical standards can address every situation. Physical therapist assistants are encouraged to seek additional advice or consultation in instances where the guidance of the Standards of Ethical Conduct may not be definitive.

Standards

Standard #1: Physical therapist assistants shall respect the inherent dignity, and rights, of all individuals.

1A. Physical therapist assistants shall act in a respectful manner toward each person regardless of age, gender, race, nationality, religion, ethnicity, social or economic status, sexual orientation, health condition, or disability.

1B. Physical therapist assistants shall recognize their personal biases and shall not discriminate against others in the provision of physical therapy services.

Standard #2: Physical therapist assistants shall be trustworthy and compassionate in addressing the rights and needs of patients/clients.

2A. Physical therapist assistants shall act in the best interests of patients/ clients over the interests of the physical therapist assistant.

2B. Physical therapist assistants shall provide physical therapy interventions with compassionate and caring behaviors that incorporate the individual and cultural differences of patients/ clients.

2C. Physical therapist assistants shall provide patients/clients with information regarding the interventions they provide.

2D. Physical therapist assistants shall protect confidential patient/client information and, in collaboration with the physical therapist, may disclose confidential information to appropriate authorities only when allowed or as required by law.

Standard #3: Physical therapist assistants shall make sound decisions in collaboration with the physical therapist and within the boundaries established by laws and regulations.

3A. Physical therapist assistants shall make objective decisions in the patient's/ client's best interest in all practice settings.

3B. Physical therapist assistants shall be guided by information about best practice regarding physical therapy interventions.

3C. Physical therapist assistants shall make decisions based upon their level of competence and consistent with patient/client values.

3D. Physical therapist assistants shall not engage in conflicts of interest that interfere with making sound decisions.

3E. Physical therapist assistants shall provide physical therapy services under the direction and supervision of a physical therapist and shall communicate with the physical therapist when patient/ client status requires modifications to the established plan of care.

Standard #4: Physical therapist assistants shall demonstrate integrity in their relationships with patients/ clients, families, colleagues, students, other health care providers, employers, payers, and the public.

4A. Physical therapist assistants shall provide truthful, accurate, and relevant information and shall not make misleading representations.

4B. Physical therapist assistants shall not exploit persons over whom they have supervisory, evaluative or other authority (e.g., patients/clients, students, supervisees, research participants, or employees).

4C. Physical therapist assistants shall discourage misconduct by health care professionals and report illegal or unethical acts to the relevant authority, when appropriate.

4D. Physical therapist assistants shall report suspected cases of abuse involving children or vulnerable adults to the supervising physical therapist and the appropriate authority, subject to law.

4E. Physical therapist assistants shall not engage in any sexual relationship with any of their patients/clients, supervisees, or students.

4F. Physical therapist assistants shall not harass anyone verbally, physically, emotionally, or sexually.

Standard #5: Physical therapist assistants shall fulfill their legal and ethical obligations.

5A. Physical therapist assistants shall comply with applicable local, state, and federal laws and regulations.

5B. Physical therapist assistants shall support the supervisory role of the physical therapist to ensure quality care and promote patient/client safety.

5C. Physical therapist assistants involved in research shall abide by accepted standards governing protection of research participants.

5D. Physical therapist assistants shall encourage colleagues with physical, psychological, or substance-related impairments that may adversely impact their professional responsibilities to seek assistance or counsel

5E. Physical therapist assistants who have knowledge that a colleague is unable to perform their professional responsibilities with reasonable skill and safety shall report this information to the appropriate authority.

Standard #6: Physical therapist assistants shall enhance their competence through the lifelong acquisition and refinement of knowledge, skills, and abilities.

6A. Physical therapist assistants shall achieve and maintain clinical competence.

6B. Physical therapist assistants shall engage in lifelong learning consistent with changes in their

roles and responsibilities and advances in the practice of physical therapy.

6C. Physical therapist assistants shall support practice environments that support career development and lifelong learning.

Standard #7: Physical therapist assistants shall support organizational behaviors and business practices that benefit patients/clients and society.

7A. Physical therapist assistants shall promote work environments that support ethical and accountable decision-making.

7B. Physical therapist assistants shall not accept gifts or other considerations that influence or give an appearance of influencing their decisions.

7C. Physical therapist assistants shall fully disclose any financial interest they have in products or services that they recommend to patients/clients.

7D. Physical therapist assistants shall ensure that documentation for their interventions accurately reflects the nature and extent of the services provided.

7E. Physical therapist assistants shall refrain from employment arrangements, or other arrangements, that prevent physical therapist assistants from fulfilling ethical obligations to patients/clients.

Standard #8: Physical therapist assistants shall participate in efforts to meet the health needs of people locally, nationally, or globally.

8A. Physical therapist assistants shall support organizations that meet the health needs of people who are economically disadvantaged, uninsured, and underinsured.

8B. Physical therapist assistants shall advocate for people with impairments, activity limitations, participation restrictions, and disabilities in order to promote their participation in community and society.

8C. Physical therapist assistants shall be responsible stewards of health care resources by collaborating with physical therapists in order to avoid overutilization or underutilization of physical therapy services.

8D. Physical therapist assistants shall educate members of the public about the benefits of physical therapy.

Appendix E

Equipment Use

Sample District Policy and Procedures for General Use of Equipment

I. Equipment

    A. A piece of equipment is identified as educationally necessary for a student, and is one whose usage needs to be monitored by a therapist.

    B. Types of equipment would include mobility, positioning, and transfer equipment such as:

        1. Stander

        2. Gait Trainer

        3. Seating Systems that include

            a. Systems that require the use of a pelvic positioning belt or other positioning straps will be included

            b. Systems that use a tray where adult assist is required will be included

        4. Wheelchair

        5. Sidelyer

        6. Mechanical Lift

II. Equipment Forms

    A. Trial Form

        1. If the therapist determines a piece of equipment may be educationally necessary, a call to the parents will be made, informing them of the trial usage. This initial contact will be documented on a form, referred to simply as the Trial Form.

        2. Once the initial trial is completed, the result of the trial will be documented on the Trial Form. The student's parents will be apprised of the trial result.

        3. Subsequent trials will be done by the therapist to determine educational necessity. The trial duration will be determined by the therapist. The results of the trials(s) will be documented on the Trial Form.

        4. If the therapist, in collaboration with the education team, determines the equipment is educationally necessary and appropriate for the student, the therapist will complete an Equipment Usage Form. The student's parents will be notified of such.

5. If the therapist, in collaboration with the education team, determines the equipment is not educationally necessary or appropriate, the use of the equipment will be discontinued. The student's parents will be notified of such.

B. Protocol for Equipment Usage

   1. The Protocol for Equipment Usage will be filled out if any of the below criteria are met:

      a. The therapist determines, after completing an equipment trial, that a piece of equipment (either district owned or personal) is educationally necessary, and requires monitoring by a therapist.

      b. The education determines that the equipment is educationally necessary and requires monitoring by a therapist.

   2. The Protocol for Equipment Usage DOES NOT need to be filled out if the student is not being monitored by a therapist, and/or the student is safe and independent with the use of their equipment.

   3. Specifics regarding transfers, supervision, and equipment settings will be put in the student's equipment binder (See Equipment Binders, section III). This binder is kept in the student's homeroom or base classroom. The Protocol for Equipment Usage will be a part of the documentation contained in the student equipment binder.

   4. Only staff trained in the use of the equipment, as documented on the Protocol for Equipment Usage, may set up the student, remove the student from the equipment, and directly supervise the student's use of the equipment.

   5. Staff may only use the equipment with the student designated on the Protocol for Equipment Usage.

C. Monthly Equipment Check Form

   1. Therapists will complete this form on a monthly basis for each piece of equipment that has a Protocol for Equipment Usage.

   2. Therapists will follow the form's directions to provide complete information.

   3. Therapists will update the Protocol for Equipment Usage, pictures in the classroom binder, and specifications in the classroom binder as they deem necessary.

D. Equipment Use Log

Educators/therapists will complete the Equipment Use Log on a daily basis or as specified on the IEP.

III. Equipment Binders

A. Therapists will maintain an equipment binder for any student they are monitoring who is using the types of equipment listed under section I.

B. The Equipment Binder will contain the following forms:

1. Trial Equipment Protocol (depending on whether a trial was completed)

2. Protocol for Equipment Usage

3. Monthly Equipment Check

4. Manufacturer's Product Information (if available)

5. Manufacturer's Maintenance Schedule

6. Pictures of the student positioned in the device, and specific recommendations regarding positioning, transfers, adjustments, settings, accessories, etc.

C. Equipment Binders will be kept on file for 2 years following transfer, dismissal from services, or graduation.

IV. IEP Documentation

A. Special Factors (DPI Form I-5) section may note information regarding the assistive technology devices and services.

B. Supplementary Aids and Services (DPI Form I-9) section may note specific information regarding transfers and functional mobility and will include amount/frequency, duration, and location of use.

C. Program Modifications and Support for Staff (DPI Form I-9) section contains specific information regarding staff training.

D. Changing Equipment Use on an Existing IEP

1. District may reconvene the IEP team to consider and document equipment changes.

2. District may contact parent for agreement to change the IEP without a meeting using DPI Forms I-10A and I-10B.

V. Equipment Maintenance

A. The therapist will instruct teachers to regularly inspect equipment and discontinue use of the device if there is a safety concern. Teachers will notify the therapist of their concerns. The therapist will inspect the equipment.

B. The therapist, as a part of a monthly inspection, will refer to the manufacture's recommended maintenance schedule. This form will be kept in a plastic sleeve in the student's Equipment Binder.

C. The therapist will mark that the equipment was inspected on the Monthly Equipment Check Form in the designated area.

D. The therapist will determine the amount and level of maintenance of equipment that he or she can perform e.g. tightening of knobs, adjustment of straps, etc. and will complete that maintenance.

E. Maintenance on district equipment that is above and beyond the ability of the therapist will be deferred to the district's Supervisor of Operations.

F. Maintenance on a student's personal equipment that is above and beyond the ability of the therapist will be deferred to the student's parents.

G. Maintenance that is above and beyond the ability of the district's maintenance staff will be deferred to the therapist and Director of Special Education. The repairs will be contracted to the appropriate company.

H. If the equipment (personal or district) is deemed unsafe upon the therapist's inspection, the item will be removed immediately. For personal equipment, the student's parents will be notified.

Kutschera, Dan. 2009. Neenah Joint School District, Neenah, WI. Adapted with Permission.

Guidelines for the Use of Weighted Blankets and Vests

- The weighted blanket is NEVER to be used as a restraint.

- Educational staff must consult with an occupational therapist before using a weighted blanket or vest with a student.

- The child's head must never be, or allowed to be, covered by the blanket.

- The child must be able to easily slip out of the blanket if he or she wishes to do so (it is not a confinement).

- A child using a weighted blanket or vest must never be unsupervised.

- A weighted blanket or vest should be approximately no more than 5% of the student's body weight.

- Staff should know about any medical considerations for the student prior to using a weighted blanket or vest.

- Use of a weighted blanket or vest should be discussed at the IEP meeting and its use should be written into the student's IEP with the parents' acknowledgement.

- Educational staff must document use of the weighted blanket and/or vest on a log. The log can be used to evaluate the effectiveness of this sensory tool.

Monthly Equipment Check

Date:_____   Equipment : _____

Student: _____ Therapist name: _____

Comments:

_____

_____

_____

_____

Teacher name: _____

Teacher concerns: ❑ Yes   ❑ No

If yes, explain

_____

_____

_____

If applicable, student comments

_____

_____

_____

❑ Equipment check completed

❑ Student absent, reschedule to _____

Changes: ❑ Yes   ❑ No

If yes, indicate change

_____

_____

_____

IF CHANGES MADE The equipment usage form must be completed.

Protocol for Equipment Usage

Student: _____ School: _____

Program: _____

Equipment: _____

Student height: _____ Student weight:_____

Student use of equipment complies with manufacturer's product recommendations in the following categories. *Check all that apply.*

    ❑ Transfer   ❑ Standing   ❑ Height/Weight   ❑ Adjustment   ❑Maintenance

Accessories: _____

_____

_____

Inspection of equipment date: _____

Inspection of equipment with student date: _____

Frequency/duration of student in equipment: _____

    ❑ Frequency/duration of student in equipment documented in IEP

Trial dates completed prior to use: _____/_____/_____/_____/_____

Proper use settings: _____

_____

_____

ATTACH Product Information

Supervision Requirements

    ❑ Adult Supervision at All Times   ❑Other…

Method of Transfer:

    ❑ One Person Transfer   ❑ Mechanical Transfer   ❑ Two Person Transfer   ❑ Other…

Staff Trained to Use	Date

Parent(s) Notified Date: _____

Therapist: _____ Date: _____

Trial Equipment Protocol

Date: _____   Program: _____

Student ID: _____   Equipment: _____

Therapist: _____   Student Height: _____

School: _____   Student Weight: _____

Student use of equipment complies with manufacturer's product recommendations in the following categories. Check all that apply and provide comments.

❏ Transfer _____

❏ Standing _____

❏ Height/Weight _____

❏ Adjustment _____

❏ Maintenance _____

Accessories: _____

_____

_____

Inspection of Equipment Date: _____   with Student Date: _____

Parents Notified Date: _____

Parents Present During Trial: _____

Date	Outcome/Notes

Attach Product Information

Method of Transfer:

❏ One Person Transfer   ❏ Mechanical Transfer

❏ Two Person Transfer   ❏ Other_____

Discontinue Use of Equipment Date: _____

❏ Continue–Complete Equipment Protocol Student Form

❏ IEP Review Date: _____

Equipment Use Log

Student	Date	Start Time	End Time	Total Time	Supervising Staff	Student Response

Appendix F

Position Descriptions

School Occupational Therapist

Nature of Position

Occupational therapists provide services to children who need special education, and to educational staff when children require occupational therapy to benefit from special education. Occupational therapists work to improve, develop, restore, or maintain a child's active participation in activities of daily living, work, leisure, and play in educational environments. Consistent with state and federal law, school occupational therapists are related service personnel.

Responsible To

Director of Special Education

Position Qualifications

1. Bachelor's, master's, or doctoral degree in occupational therapy from a school accredited by the American Occupational Therapy Association Accreditation Council for Occupational Therapy Education
2. Initial certification from the National Board for Certification in Occupational Therapy
3. Current occupational therapist license from the Wisconsin Department of Regulation and Licensing, Occupational Therapy Affiliated Credentialing Board. Current occupational therapist license (812) from the Wisconsin Department of Public Instruction.

Goals and Responsibilities

1. **Identification and planning.** The occupational therapist evaluates children, interprets evaluation findings as a member of the Individualized Education Program (IEP) team, and plans appropriate intervention.
2. **Intervention.** The occupational therapist develops and implements direct and indirect services based on individual evaluation and the IEP. The focus of these services may include but are not limited to a child's
    *   activities of daily living
    *   work and productive activities
    *   play or leisure activities
    *   sensorimotor components of performance
    *   cognitive integration and cognitive components of performance
    *   psychosocial skills and psychological components of performance
3. **Program administration and management.** The occupational therapist participates in the local education agency's comprehensive planning process for the education of children with exceptional educational needs. The occupational therapist works with the director of special education to establish the procedures for implementing the occupational therapy service. The occupational therapist may supervise occupational therapy assistants.

4. **Community awareness.** The occupational therapist provides information for administrators, school personnel, parents, and non-school agencies regarding school occupational therapy.

5. **Professional growth and ethics.** The occupational therapist adheres to the ethical standards of the profession and participates in professional growth activities and continuing education opportunities. The occupational therapist adheres to established rules, regulations and laws, and works cooperatively to accomplish the goals and objectives of the local education agency.

Essential Job Functions

The occupational therapist performs the following position functions, as the school district requires:

1. Conduct appropriate evaluations of children referred for suspected disabilities and prepare written reports of the evaluations conducted and the findings.
2. Participate in meetings as a member of the IEP team.
3. Participate in the development of IEPs for children found to have disabilities.
4. Provide direct and indirect occupational therapy to children with disabilities in educational environments.
5. Collaborate with other school personnel regarding occupational therapy and the children's needs.
6. Travel to and among schools to provide services to children.
7. Maintain records of service provided.
8. Transfer and position children and equipment with assistance as necessary to provide occupational therapy.

School Occupational Therapy Assistant

Nature of Position
Occupational therapy assistants provide services to children with disabilities and to educational staff under the supervision of an occupational therapist when children require occupational therapy to benefit from special education. Occupational therapy assistants follow a treatment plan developed by the occupational therapist and work to improve, develop, restore, or maintain a child's active participation in activities of daily living, work, leisure and play in educational environments. Consistent with state and federal law, school occupational therapy assistants are related service personnel.

Responsible To
Director of Special Education; professionally under the supervision of a DPI licensed occupational therapist.

Position Qualifications
1. Associate degree as an occupational therapy assistant from a school accredited by the American Occupational Therapy Association Accreditation Council for Occupational Therapy Education
2. Initial certification from the National Board for Certification in Occupational Therapy
3. Current occupational therapy assistant license from the Wisconsin Department of Regulation and Licensing, Occupational Therapy Affiliated Credentialing Board
4. Current school occupational therapy assistant license (885) from the Wisconsin Department of Public Instruction

Goals and Responsibilities
1. **Intervention.** The occupational therapy assistant provides quality occupational therapy services to children with disabilities, which an occupational therapist delegates and supervises. The occupational therapist determines the level of supervision based on the occupational therapy assistant's education, experience, and service competency. Under close or general supervision, the occupational therapy assistant

   - assists with data collection and evaluation.
   - provides direct service according to a written treatment plan that the occupational therapist develops alone or with the occupational therapy assistant.
   - recommends modification of treatment approaches to the occupational therapist to reflect the child's changing needs.
   - adapts environments, tools, materials, and activities according to the child's needs.
   - communicates and interacts with other team members, school personnel and families in collaboration with an occupational therapist.
   - maintains treatment areas, equipment and supply inventory as the service plan requires.
   - maintains records and documentation as the service plan requires.
   - participates in the development of policies and procedures in collaboration with an occupational therapist.

2. **Community awareness.** The occupational therapy assistant provides information for administrators, school personnel, parents, and non-school agencies regarding school occupational therapy.

3. **Professional growth and ethics.** The occupational therapy assistant adheres to the ethical standards of the profession and participates in professional growth activities and continuing education opportunities. The occupational therapy assistant adheres to established rules, regulations and laws, and works cooperatively to accomplish the goals and objectives of the local education agency.

Essential Job Functions

The occupational therapy assistant performs the following position functions, as the school district requires and which the occupational therapist delegates and supervises:

1. Assist with evaluations of children referred for possible disabilities.
2. Provide direct and indirect occupational therapy to children with disabilities in educational environments.
3. Assist the occupational therapist in the provision of occupational therapy.
4. Provide information to other school personnel regarding occupational therapy and the children's needs.
5. Travel to and among schools to provide services to children.
6. Maintain records of service provided.
7. Transfer and position children as necessary to provide occupational therapy.
8. Prepare equipment and supplies as necessary for interventions.

School Physical Therapist

Nature of Position
Physical therapists provide services to children with disabilities and to educational staff when children require physical therapy to benefit from special education.

Responsible To
Director of Special Education

Position Qualifications
1. Bachelor's or master's degree in physical therapy or doctor of physical therapy from a school approved by the Physical Therapy Examining Board.
2. Current license from the Physical Therapy Examining Board
3. Current physical therapy license (817) from the Wisconsin Department of Public Instruction

Goals and Responsibilities
1. **Identification and planning.** The physical therapist evaluates children, interprets evaluation findings as a member of the Individualized Education Program (IEP) team, and plans appropriate intervention as a participant in the IEP team meeting.
2. **Intervention.** The physical therapist develops and implements direct and indirect services based on individual evaluation and the IEP. The focus of these services may include but are not limited to a child's

   - mobility, balance, coordination.
   - activity performance of motor tasks.
   - performance of transfers.
   - use of assistive, orthotic, prosthetic, adaptive, and protective devices.
   - aerobic endurance.
3. **Program administration and management.** The physical therapist participates in the local education agency's comprehensive planning process for the education of children with disabilities. The physical therapist works with the director of special education to establish the procedures for implementing physical therapy and participates in the maintenance and expansion of the physical therapy service. The physical therapist may supervise physical therapist assistants.
4. **Community awareness.** The physical therapist provides information for administrators, school personnel, parents, and non-school agencies regarding physical therapy.
5. **Professional growth and ethics.** The physical therapist adheres to the ethical standards of the profession and participates in professional growth activities and continuing education opportunities. The physical therapist adheres to established rules, regulations and laws, and works cooperatively to accomplish the goals and objectives of the local education agency.

Essential Job Functions

The physical therapist performs the following position functions, as the school district requires:

1. Conduct appropriate evaluations of children referred for special education and prepare required documentation.
2. Participate in IEP meetings.
3. Participate in the development of IEPs for children with disabilities.
4. Develop a physical therapy treatment plan for the child.
5. Provide direct and indirect physical therapy to children with disabilities.
6. Collaborate with other school personnel regarding physical therapy and the children's needs.
7. Travel to and among schools to provide services to children.
8. Maintain records of service provided.
9. Lift, transfer, and position children and equipment as necessary to provide physical therapy.

School Physical Therapist Assistant

Nature of Position
Physical therapist assistants provide physical therapy to children with disabilities under the direction and supervision of a physical therapist.

Responsible To
Director of Special Education; professionally under the supervision of a DPI licensed physical therapist.

Position Qualifications
1. Graduate of a physical therapist assistant associate degree program accredited by an agency approved by the Physical Therapy Examining Board.
2. Current physical therapist assistant license from the Physical Therapy Examining Board
3. Current school physical therapist assistant license (886) from the Wisconsin Department of Public Instruction.

Goals and Responsibilities
1. **Intervention.** The physical therapist assistant provides quality physical therapy services to children with disabilities, which a physical therapist delegates and supervises. The physical therapist assistant provides selected components of a child's physical therapy treatment plan developed by the physical therapist. The physical therapist determines the level of supervision based on the physical therapist assistant's education, training, experience, and skill level.
2. **Community awareness.** The physical therapist assistant provides information for administrators, school personnel, parents, and non-school agencies regarding physical therapy.
3. **Professional growth and ethics.** The physical therapist assistant adheres to the ethical standards of the profession and participates in professional growth activities and continuing education opportunities. The physical therapist assistant adheres to established rules, regulations and laws, and works cooperatively to accomplish the goals and objectives of the local education agency.

Essential Job Functions
The physical therapist assistant performs the following position functions, as the school district requires and which the physical therapist delegates and supervises:
1. Provides selected components of physical therapy intervention.
2. Makes modifications in interventions as directed by the physical therapist or to ensure the student's safety.
3. Lifts, transfers, and positions children and equipment as necessary to provide physical therapy.
4. Documents interventions performed, data collected, student progress, equipment provided, and communication with others.
5. Interacts with the child, family, or community providers.
6. Participates with the physical therapist in training support staff and teachers.
7. Assists in the design and fabrication of equipment or adaptations for specific children.
8. Participates in the development of policies and procedures.
9. Helps with budget development, ordering equipment and supplies.
10. Participates in discussions regarding schedules and assignment of children.
11. Travels to and among schools to provide services to children.
12. Assists with maintenance of inventory and records.